T0180064

Fundamentals of
Transference-Focused
Psychotherapy

Richard G. Hersh • Eve Caligor
Frank E. Yeomans

Fundamentals of Transference-Focused Psychotherapy

Applications in Psychiatric and Medical Settings

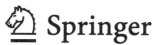 Springer

Richard G. Hersh
Department of Psychiatry,
  Columbia University College
  of Physicians and Surgeons
Columbia University Center for
  Psychoanalytic Training and
  Research
New York, NY, USA

Eve Caligor
Department of Psychiatry,
  Columbia University College
  of Physicians and Surgeons
Columbia University Center for
  Psychoanalytic Training and
  Research
New York, NY, USA

Frank E. Yeomans
Department of Psychiatry,
  Weill Cornell Medical Center
Columbia University Center for
  Psychoanalytic Training and
  Research
New York, NY, USA

ISBN 978-3-319-82980-7   ISBN 978-3-319-44091-0   (eBook)
DOI 10.1007/978-3-319-44091-0

Printed on acid-free paper

This Springer imprint is published by Springer Nature
The registered company is Springer International Publishing AG
The registered company address is: Gewerbestrasse 11, 6330 Cham, Switzerland

Preface

Transference-focused psychotherapy (TFP) had its clinical origins on the campus of New York-Presbyterian Hospital, Westchester Division, in 1980. Under the leadership of John Oldham and John Clarkin, Otto Kernberg and senior psychiatrists in the department met on a regular basis to view and discuss videotaped sessions of their individual treatment with borderline patients. It was a bottom-up approach: we viewed the sessions with an eye to what the clinician was doing in the treatment in order to generalize to principles of intervention with these intriguing, quite disturbed, and difficult to treat patients. The goal was to generate a description at the level of principles to inform a psychodynamic treatment based on object relations theory of borderline personality disorder (BPD) patients.

In order to empirically investigate the impact of TFP, a written manual describing the treatment was a necessary tool to enable replication of any results. An eminent psychiatrist in the department, Dr. Gerald Klerman, had "manualized" interpersonal therapy (IPT) and was consulted about how to devise a TFP treatment manual. He suggested that strategies and techniques of the treatment be carefully explained and illustrated with clinical vignettes. His advice was to continue articulating treatment techniques illustrated with clinical vignettes until the treatment was fully described.

This preparation enabled us to apply and receive an NIMH treatment development grant to generate initial effect sizes of TFP. With encouraging results, two randomized clinical trials of TFP have contributed to our knowledge of its impact on borderline patients. Throughout this process, we continued to observe actual treatment sessions, and modify and improve the treatment. A succession of treatment manuals (Clarkin, Yeomans, & Kernberg, 1999; Clarkin, Yeomans and Kernberg, 2006; Yeomans, Clarkin & Kernberg, 2015) documents the modifications in the treatment as our experience grew. Observation of clinical cases, articulation of difficulties and solutions, and re-articulation of the treatment are an iterative and enriching approach.

Now with this volume, Richard Hersh, Eve Caligor, and Frank Yeomans have taken us to the next level by demonstrating how the principles of TFP can be adapted to different patient groups and different treatment settings. This is a rich, clinically-based approach utilizing the principles of TFP flexibly and creatively with patients across a spectrum of personality difficulties and symptomatic pictures. This next step in establishing an approach of "applied TFP" should bring the critical concepts and clinical techniques of this treatment to a wider audience. There are simply not enough clinicians trained in the evidence-based therapies for borderline personality disorder and the other severe personality disorder presentations. While we continue to refine our approach as an extended individual psychotherapy, "applied TFP" allows us to bring our experience and insights into a broader sphere, fulfilling a crucial public health role informed, as noted, by our bottom-up approach.

John F. Clarkin, Ph.D.
Codirector, Personality Disorders Institute,
Weill Cornell Medical Center
Clinical Professor of Psychology in Psychiatry,
Weill Cornell Medical Center
New York, NY, USA

Contents

Chapter 1
Transference-Focused Psychotherapy (TFP) and Its Applications: Introduction to TFP and the Roles of the Structural Interview, Goal Setting, and Contracting

1. *TFP's origins are steeped in traditional psychoanalytic object relations theory and practice, but its key concepts should have wide appeal to contemporary clinicians, including those without specialized training, in a variety of treatment situations.*
2. *The structural interview is the cornerstone of the TFP approach and has utility as a step required for TFP as an individual psychotherapy and as an assessment process to be used more broadly.*
3. *TFP emphasizes a deliberate, detailed process of identifying the patient's personal goals and treatment goals, an orienting intervention for patient and therapist, and a requirement for effectiveness in this particular psychotherapy.*
4. *TFP prioritizes the treatment contract, the bedrock of the treatment frame, as an irreducible anchor of this psychotherapy process, requiring persistent engagement over time by both therapist and patient.*

© Springer International Publishing Switzerland 2016   1
R.G. Hersh et al., *Fundamentals of Transference-Focused Psychotherapy*, DOI 10.1007/978-3-319-44091-0_1

1.1   Introduction

Transference-focused psychotherapy (TFP) is a specific treatment developed over many years for a specific patient population – individuals with borderline personality disorder (BPD). TFP is a manualized treatment (meaning clinicians are guided by a detailed treatment manual outlining the approach to treatment) and evidence-based (meaning it has been studied and compared to other treatment interventions for the same patient population). TFP has been shown to be effective in multiple domains: retention in treatment (patients staying engaged in psychotherapy vs. dropping out early), suicidal and self-injurious behavior (including the number of self-harm attempts and the medical severity of these attempts), self-reports of symptoms (a reduction of suicidal ideation, depression, and anxiety), and social adjustment (positive changes in friendship and work) [1–3]. This accumulated data supports TFP as an individual psychotherapy for a particular patient population; numerous studies and textbooks have been published on this subject. *The goal of this book is to further extend the influence of TFP theory and practice by introducing TFP as a way of thinking about and treating patients beyond a limited group (patients with BPD by DSM-5 criteria) and beyond a particular treatment modality (extended individual psychotherapy) for which it was developed.*

Who are the clinicians who can use TFP principles in their work, and what are the clinical situations where TFP principles can be useful in patient care? The answer to this question begins with consideration of who the clinicians are in the mental health and medical fields treating patients with significant personality disorder (PD) pathology. The answer is almost all clinicians seeing adolescent and adult patients. Are there exceptions? To be sure, clinicians treating only young children, or those patients with primary psychotic disorders or dementia, for example, would be in this category. That said, patients with PD pathology are well represented in almost all mental health settings and in many general medical settings as well [4, 5]. Certainly, many, if not most, psychiatrists, psychologists, and social workers will encounter PD patients in their careers. All clinicians working in adult psychiatric inpatient settings and emergency rooms will have the experience of evaluating and treating PD patients. Studies indicate that clinicians in most direct-care medical fields will interface with patients with PD symptomatology at relatively high rates as well [6]. The bottom line: patients with serious PD pathology will present for care in a wide variety of settings, for a variety of reasons (not limited to PD complaints), to a wide range of clinicians.

The application of TFP principles begins with the process of clinical assessment. TFP as an individual psychotherapy stresses the advantage of the structural interview, a comprehensive and intuitive way of evaluating patients [7, 8]. Clearly not every clinician will have the time or inclination to complete the structural interview as it is designed; key elements of the structural interview, however, can be incorporated into even the briefest patient evaluation process. The structural interview asks not only whether a patient fits into one or more diagnostic categories but also, more generally, how does this patient function in the key areas of his or her life? The structural interview prompts the evaluating clinician to ask questions that will begin to clarify (1) what might be the best treatment for the complaint at hand, (2) the prospective patient's overall prognosis, and (3) how might I best gear my interaction with this patient.

An individual TFP treatment is anchored by an explicit discussion of a patient's personal goals and treatment goals. It may seem unnecessary to stress this point; after all, aren't all treatments premised on clearly defined goals? Yet experience with patients with severe PD presentations suggests that it is easy for a patient and treater to fall into a desultory pattern, divorced from a defined treatment focus, when *being in the treatment* becomes more important than *where the treatment is heading*. A TFP approach will ask: what are the patient's personal goals related to studies, work, or relationships? In terms of treatment goals, such an inquiry would explore how any particular psychotherapy might help a patient with targeted symptoms. While TFP itself is premised on clearly defined and orienting personal and treatment goals, one possible outcome of a clinician's evaluation using the structural interview might be to recommend a treatment that is more supportive (and less exploratory) than TFP. The very act of asking a patient about personal and treatment goals can be a powerful antidote to a commonly observed phenomenon – the patient with a PD diagnosis who consciously or unconsciously experiences treatment as *something done to him or her by another person,* and not a collaborative experience, initiated and continued at the behest of the patient.

TFP stresses the paramount importance of the treatment frame. The frame is the set of mutually agreed-upon details of the treatment arrangement, everything from the expected issues of scheduling and billing, to more fraught areas of discussion, such as crisis management or hospitalization. In TFP the treatment frame is the end result of the purposeful and frank contracting process. The contracting process in TFP takes as long as it needs to; it is not rushed or routine, and a contracting process that is free of some degree of friction or push-back by the patient is likely to be superficial, without a thoughtful engagement on the part of the patient. The contracting process has simultaneous goals: to create a safe and comfortable treatment situation for both the patient and the therapist *and* to serve as a likely dress rehearsal for what is to come in the therapy. A dress rehearsal for what? The "transference" in transference-focused psychotherapy is the patient's total experience of the therapist, filtered through the prism of the patient's history, experience of others, and current state of mind. This view is based on the idea that personality is fundamentally a person's way of processing all the data coming from the world around him and that an individual patient's "processing system" can be observed in the interaction with the therapist. The therapist expects to observe revealing responses by the patient in the introduction of the contract – paranoid and angry or agreeable and idealizing are two possible responses among many. The contracting process and associated treatment frame are put into place to facilitate the expression of this transference and the patient and therapist's collaboration in dissection of this transference over time. The introduction of a contracting process and the establishment of a treatment frame are not, by definition, restricted to an individual psychotherapy. Clinicians of all kinds can benefit from establishing ground rules at the start of any treatment relationship. After all, if the clinician doesn't feel comfortable or safe, how can he or she provide a high quality of care?

1.2   An Overview of TFP Treatment

- *TFP is a treatment with roots in psychoanalytic tradition and object relation theory, but with critical adjustments tailored to accommodate a specific group of patients with severe personality disorder pathology.*
- *TFP is guided by a detailed treatment manual, and accumulated research supports its status as an evidence-based treatment for BPD.*
- *TFP's overarching theoretical framework and clinical interventions have certain essential differences that distinguish it from more familiar supportive and cognitive-behavioral approaches.*
- *"Applied TFP" uses fundamental TFP concepts and interventions in varied clinical situations, distinct from the originally investigated individual psychotherapy treatment format.*

The term "transference-focused psychotherapy" might suggest to some of today's mental health or medical clinicians, particularly those who are not versed in contemporary psychoanalytic theory and practice, an "old school" or even fusty treatment modality, suited to a past era, and now either inaccessible or irrelevant. This would be an unfortunate and inaccurate conclusion. The era when psychoanalytic thinking wholly dominated the treatment of individuals with personality disorder pathology, with highly variable success, is long past; TFP should not be seen as a last-gasp vestige of this era. In fact, TFP is a state-of-the art, manualized, and empirically supported psychodynamically-informed individual psychotherapy treatment for patients with borderline personality disorder (BPD), one demonstrated to be of important utility for this substantial patient population with notably high rates of morbidity and mortality [9].

As noted, TFP was developed as a treatment for BPD, and TFP research studies have focused exclusively on patients with BPD. BPD is a common psychiatric disorder, as reflected in community studies (with rates of approximately 2 % or the population, *significantly higher* than that of schizophrenia), well represented in inpatient and outpatient population samples (studies suggest 20 % of psychiatric inpatient and 10 % of psychiatric outpatients meet criteria for BPD), and likely widely *underdiagnosed* (as reflected in studies showing that clinicians evaluating patients with structured interviews are significantly more likely to make a BPD diagnosis than those clinicians assessing patients without specific prompts that might yield a PD diagnosis) [10–14]. BPD is, therefore, (1) common, (2) likely underdiagnosed, and (3) very clearly associated with high use of almost all psychiatric services including hospitalizations, outpatient psychotherapy, and medications [15]. On top of that, BPD has a relatively high rate of completed suicide (somewhere between 6 and 10 %), making treatment of patients with BPD understandably a source of care and concern for most treaters [16].

TFP is one of a group of evidence-based treatments for BPD that includes: dialectical behavior therapy (DBT), good psychiatric management (GPM), supportive psychotherapy (SPT), mentalization-based therapy (MBT), schema-focused therapy (SFT), and the STEPPS intervention [17]. Even with this proliferation of evidence-based treatments for BPD, the demand for clinicians able to treat patients with BPD and other serious personality disorders will likely outstrip the supply of suitably trained clinicians for years, if not decades, to come, contributing to a genuine, if underappreciated, public health crisis [18]. To this end, the first two chapters of this book have as their focus: (1) the essential elements of TFP offered as an individual psychotherapy for patients with severe personality disorder pathology (including, but not limited to, borderline personality disorder) and (2) an introduction to "applied TFP" or a collection of useful observations and practical interventions derived from TFP and appropriate for clinicians of varying levels of training, in multiple spheres, treating a mix of patients. One leader in the field, John Gunderson, described TFP as the "hardest to learn" of the evidence-based BPD treatments that helps the most challenging cases; while this may be true, "applied TFP" principles should be readily accessible to and easily employed by clinicians of differing training backgrounds and levels of experience [19].

The vast majority of research done on patients with personality disorder pathology has been done on females with BPD since the large majority of BPD patients in clinical settings are women. The treatments listed above were developed because of the serious need to employ evidence-based treatments for the most symptomatic of this population. TFP was developed in the same spirit, to aid clinicians treating the most impaired of this group of patients. TFP can be thought of as one of this list of evidence-based treatments with, for the most part, certain commonalities: a clear treatment frame, attention to affect, a focus on the treatment relationship, use of exploratory interventions, and an active therapist [20]. TFP can also be appreciated for its utility more broadly as a way to think about a variety of patients, beyond the group meeting DSM-5 criteria for BPD, and as a treatment modality for this broader group of patients, although research comparable to that available for the use of TFP for BPD has yet to be done. Who are the patients in this broader group who may benefit from a TFP approach? This chapter will review the concept of borderline *organization*, a category encompassing patients with BPD, as well as many patients meeting DSM-5 diagnostic criteria for dependent, narcissistic, histrionic, schizoid, or schizotypal personality disorders, as well as patients with personality disorder diagnoses – sadomasochistic, hypochondriacal, or hypomanic – not part of DSM-5 terminology. TFP gives clinicians a way to think about and treat a larger and more heterogeneous group than is customarily identified as likely to benefit from one of the evidence-based treatments for BPD.

TFP builds on the work of Otto Kernberg and his colleagues at the Personality Disorders Institute of the Weill Cornell Medical College, contributing to a robust literature on an approach to treating patients with personality disorder pathology informed by object relations theory. As noted, Kernberg and his colleagues have authored essential papers and texts, including the TFP manual (Transference-Focused Psychotherapy for Borderline Personality Disorder: A Clinical Guide, by Yeomans et al. [9], and a companion volume on the treatment of adults with higher level personality pathology (Dynamic Psychotherapy for Higher Level Personality Disorder Patients, by Caligor et al. [21], with a volume planned on the treatment of adolescent BPD patients [22], conveying the central elements of the treatment to clinicians motivated to use this intervention in individual psychotherapy. This book is not meant as a substitute for the TFP manual and its companion volumes, but rather an extension of its core principles for use by a broader audience of therapists in different fields.

The purpose of the introductory chapters of this volume is to systematically take apart the key elements of this treatment in a way that makes these elements accessible for clinicians of all kinds and to consider how many of these elements on their own may be useful to clinicians who are *not* conducting an extended individual psychotherapy, but can nevertheless benefit from applying TFP concepts in the work they do.

This chapter includes a glossary of terms frequently used in the TFP literature; terms highlighted below in **bold** are among those listed in the glossary.

TFP as a manualized individual treatment has a clearly delineated approach. The essential steps include:

Getting Started

1. A thorough assessment process using the **structural interview**.
2. An appreciation of functioning in multiple spheres informing consideration about a patient's **level of personality organization** and prognosis.
3. The clinician's active monitoring of **three channels of communication:** what the patient says, how the patients acts, and how the therapist feels.
4. Appreciation of the admixture of **repression-based defenses** and **splitting-based defenses** a patient exhibits.
5. Elucidation of a patient's personal goals and treatment goals.
6. An extended process of contracting, leading to the establishment of a living **treatment frame,** tailored to the specific pathology of, and expected challenges from, the individual patient.

When the Treatment Begins

7. Managing the likely initial confusion associated with severe PD pathology by **"naming the actors"** involved in the moment-to-moment interaction between patient and therapist to help contain the patient and orient the therapist. In more technical terms, this is identifying the **object relations dyads** that emerge in treatment.
8. Identification of moments when the roles within the dominant **object relations dyads** reverse, or a **role reversal.** This helps patients see aspects of their personality they tend to see in others but not in themselves.

(continued)

(continued)

9. The therapist's efforts to maintain a stance of concern that reflects **technical neutrality** in relation to the internal conflicts the patient struggles with, with deviations from this stance when required.
10. Ongoing attention to the treatment frame, with periodic adjustments to the frame as necessary, given likely challenges from the patient.

What Happens Minute by Minute

11. The therapist's attempt to identify the content with **affective dominance** in a session (i.e., the material that has the highest emotional charge).
12. The therapist proceeding from what is most accessible to the patient's awareness to that which is less accessible (a **surface-to-depth** approach).
13. The specific techniques of **clarification, confrontation, and interpretation**, used repeatedly.
14. The therapist's orientation to the chronic, baseline (usually paranoid/fearful of others) transference in early phases of treatment.
15. Assessment of a patient's response to interpretations offered by the therapist and the meaning of this back and forth in the context of the treatment relationship.

What Happens Over Time

16. Diminishing chaos in the patient's external life, increased affect in the treatment.
17. Adjustments in the frame/contract as needed.
18. A change from a chronic paranoid transference to one with elements reflecting a more nuanced

(continued)

(continued)

experience of the therapist (and others in the patient's life) with increasing trust.

19. The therapist's appreciation of the interplay between dyads (relationship paradigms carrying different emotions).

20. The patient's gradual move from the **paranoid position** (projection of negative emotions) to the **depressive position** (taking ownership of negative emotions with the capacity for feelings of guilt) reflecting integration of previously "split" representations of self and other as totally good or bad.

Since TFP is a contemporary development of traditional psychoanalytic practice, specifically object relations theory, how could its essential elements be of use to clinicians in contemporary practice who may have limited interest in, if not outright skepticism about, psychoanalysis as they know it? TFP differs from psychoanalytic treatment in a number of fundamental ways. TFP is designed to be conducted twice weekly (rarely, if ever, with more frequency), sitting up (TFP does not use the analytic couch), and oriented toward specific, well-described personal and treatment goals (not a more general goal of "self-knowledge"). TFP is resolutely focused on the here and now; exploration of a patient's childhood or family or origin may become relevant in the treatment over time, but never at the expense of what is happening in the treatment in real time and the realities of the patient's life outside of treatment, meaning the nature and quality of the patient's studies, work, relationships, and place in the community.

An extended discussion of objects relations theory and its place in psychoanalytic thinking is beyond the scope of this book. Most clinicians are familiar with treatment approaches based on (1) supportive techniques or (2) cognitive-behavioral interventions, having had only a limited exposure to psychoanalytic theory and practice. They may understand psychoanalytic theory as premised on exploration of what is partially or fully unconscious for the patient–that symptoms or conflicts are "compromises" between underlying drives/ desires and internal or social prohibitions. (The classic example would be symptoms of anxiety that emerge from the conflict between competitive strivings and a fear of being aggressive.) TFP was developed for patients with severe personality disorder pathology because the standard psychoanalytic approach of exploring unconscious conflicts alone did not seem to work as it did with less severely disturbed patients. Object relations theory describes the individual's experience of self and other and the associated feelings (in object relations terminology the "representation of self" and the "representation of the object" connected by an affect) making up the object relations dyad. These experiences of self and other are the building blocks of personality or sense of self. For patients with severe personality disorder pathology, the problem was not simply that the origins of certain conflicts were outside the patient's awareness; the patient can be *aware* of certain feelings, but the patient is subject to momentary shifts, feeling positively, say, about a particular person or themselves, only to rapidly shift to a wholly negative experience – radical shifts, but in the patient's awareness nevertheless. The "splitting" so often referenced in discussion of borderline pathology originates, in object relations theory, with the unconscious separation of object relations dyads (the wholly positive or wholly negative sense of self or other) that are themselves in the patient's awareness as they are occurring, to some degree, although at different times.

How would TFP with its object relations orientation differ from a more familiar supportive or cognitive-behavioral approach? It may be useful to consider the same clinical situation from the three different perspectives. Let's take the example of Ms. F., a woman with BPD with a pattern of becoming easily attached to friends, invariably leading to a highly emotional rupture in the friendship when Ms. F. feels mistreated or ignored.

- The supportive psychotherapist aims to give Ms. F. advice about how to keep friends. She praises Ms. F. for the pleasing parts of her personality and attempts to engage Ms. F. in developing practical strategies when she feels distressed, like taking a warm bath or calling her sister.
- The cognitive-behavioral therapist intends to engage Ms. F. in exploration of her "faulty thinking patterns" during periods of distress. The therapist enlists Ms. F. to keep a diary card in an effort to chart together the development of her intense anger, to assess for "triggers," and to learn strategies for reframing her negative thoughts as they mount.
- The TFP therapist approaches Ms. F.'s difficulties with awareness that it may not be possible to accurately and objectively assess what, in fact, goes on with Ms. F. and her friends. The TFP therapist has the aim of setting up a frame that would allow Ms. F.'s dynamics to emerge *in the transference* (the relationship with the therapist). If they repeat the pattern Ms. F. describes in her "outside" relations, the TFP therapist has the goal of helping the patient understand what she "reads into" relations and increasing her capacity for reflection by examining together what has occurred in their relationship.

Is familiarity with psychoanalytic thinking or training in psychoanalysis a prerequisite for TFP training? It is not. The basic principles of TFP should be widely accessible, and the treatment manual does not presuppose advanced training in psychodynamic psychotherapy or psychoanalysis. As explained in the manual, TFP as an individual psychotherapy has a set of specific *strategies* (the overarching objectives of the treatment), *tactics* (the therapist's setting the secure conditions of treatment and choosing the focus with each session), and *techniques* (the therapist's minute-to-minute interventions). "Applied TFP" in this book extends the use of TFP principles to clinical situations beyond individual psychotherapy treatment to include:

- General crisis management
- Family interventions
- Inpatient psychiatric treatment
- Psychopharmacology
- Management of medical care
- Psychiatry residency training

1.3   The Structural Interview

- *The structural interview has the goal of collecting all the information that would be pursued in a standard psychiatric interview, with additional questioning to explore more fully specific areas of the patient's functioning.*
- *The structural interview follows a "circular" approach, with a focus on the interviewer's exploration of inconsistencies or points of confusion, rather than a standard "decision-tree" approach.*
- *The structural interview aims to clarify a patient's diagnosis by category but also to appraise a patient's functioning in multiple spheres, described as the patient's level of organization.*
- *The structural interview will explore elements of the standard "social history" in greater depth than is customary, with a particular focus on friendships, romance, work history, and finances.*

The standard psychiatric interview approaches data collection in a straightforward manner; the clinician uses DSM-5 diagnostic criteria as a guide and proceeds in a "decision-tree" manner, asking yes/no questions, attempting to quantify positive responses (How many panic attack symptoms? How long has the depressed patient experienced anhedonia?). This "decision-tree" approach is often extended to assessment of personality disorder symptoms, using the DSM-5 diagnostic category criteria as a guide. In recent years, there has been a movement to shift from a purely categorical approach to personality disorder diagnosis (Does the patient describe the requisite number of symptoms to meet the determined cutoff?) to a hybrid model that includes both evaluation of diagnostic category criteria *and* consideration of dimensions of personality traits (assessing the patient's level of well-being or impairment in a certain area as measured on a continuum). While this hybrid model remains part of the DSM-5 appendix, the structural interview pursues the same objective – assessment of both the particular subtype of personality traits that are in evidence and how well-functioning or impaired a particular individual might be in important ways.

With this in mind, the structural interview begins with inquiry about a patient's symptoms and history, as would be done in a standard interview, as well as investigation of the patient's self-conception and experience of others. The structural interview process addresses first any complaints or observable symptoms that might reflect a primary organic presentation (meaning medical or physical in origin) or major psychiatric disorder that might either preclude or strongly affect an exploratory psychotherapy process. Once these processes have been assessed and ruled out, the structural interview then moves on to the phase that asks the patient to describe himself or herself and asks the patient to describe one or two people with whom he or she has a close relationship. The structural interview has a distinct rhythm; the questioner will repeatedly circle back to any area of confusion or inconsistency in the patient's story. The questioner will also expand the often neglected social history component of the evaluation process, in an effort to gage the patient's functioning in important areas, questions about school or work and the nature of relationships with friends, spouses, children, and parents, for example.

The TFP therapist using the structural interview has the goal of assessing the patient in multiple spheres that can be recalled with the mnemonic RADIOS:

Reality testing
Aggression
Defenses
Identify diffusion/consolidation
Object relations
Superego or moral values

These six areas of exploration of the structural interview aid the TFP therapist to move beyond the process of generating a differential diagnosis using DSM-5 categories only. This process of investigation allows the TFP therapist to consider: How well-functioning or impaired is this particular patient in a number of key areas of his or her life? What can I learn in the assessment phase to help me guide this patient to the appropriate treatment targeting a primarily biological/organic problem or targeting a more complex combination of biology and psychological organization? How should I discuss my understanding of the patient's difficulties with him/her? And, how can I begin to determine the patient's prognosis?

Reality Testing: The structural interview has a goal of exploring the patient's capacity for reality testing in part to assess for the appropriateness of a referral for exploratory treatment. The structural interview aims to clarify a patient's degree of persistent frank psychotic thinking (an exclusion criteria for TFP), transient psychosis under stress (expected in some BPD patients, with the potential for compromising the capacity to use exploratory treatment), and an overall social inappropriateness (often a source of concern, e.g., in the treatment of patients with schizotypal personality disorder). The TFP classification of personality disorders combining categorical and dimensional constructs identifies impairment in reality testing as consistent with the lower borderline or psychotic organization, i.e., the more severely impaired patients. However, patients at the borderline level of personality disorder in general have a fragility of reality testing based on the imposition of an internal mental representation on their objective reality (e.g., "You looked at the clock, so you must want to get rid of me.")

Aggression: The TFP approach places significant emphasis on the assessment of a patient's level of aggressive affects and in particular the expression of ego-syntonic aggression. The identification of marked aggression in any patient will cue the therapist to consider the way this trait might undermine the treatment, informing prognosis. TFP clinicians are particularly sensitive to patients presenting with ego-syntonic aggression, paranoia, antisocial traits, and narcissistic personality disorder symptoms – a syndrome described as "malignant narcissism" with a particular (poor) prognosis and distinct requirements (an unusually rigorous treatment frame) for effective treatment.

Defenses: The TFP approach places much weight on the evaluation of a patient's predominant defenses and the relative contributions of splitting-based defenses and repression-based defenses. Defenses are the patient's partially or fully unconscious ways of negotiating conflicting impulses, prohibitions, and the realities of everyday life. The central distinction between repression-based vs. splitting-based defenses is at the heart of the TFP understanding of severe personality disorder pathology and is considered a critical marker in determining personality organization. Repression-based defenses follow the psychoanalytic understanding of the ways conflictual material can lead a patient to keep certain difficult thoughts or feeling out of awareness in a consistent way. The typical repression-based defenses – repression, isolation of affect, reaction formation, and intellectualization – allow the patient to manage situations when these repressed feelings come close to entering awareness. These are considered more "mature" defenses, allowing generally for more relative flexibility and adaptive functioning. Splitting-based defenses do not presuppose evenly repressed material but rather suggest a set of coping strategies marked by keeping separate "all good" feelings from "all bad" feelings. The splitting-based defenses include: alternating idealization and devaluation, denial, projection, projective identification, and omnipotent control. While these defenses provide some relief from the anxiety of psychological conflict, they are relatively maladaptive since they introduce a greater degree of rigidity into personality functioning and interacting with the world than do repression-based defenses. When conducting the structural interview, the clinician is alert to evidence of patterns of defensive operation. As noted, patients will use a mix of defenses, determined by psychosocial stressors at a given time.

Identity Diffusion vs. Consolidation: Considered the single most important area of consideration for the therapist conducting an evaluation using the structural interview, the measure of identity diffusion vs. consolidation gages the patient's degree of consistency and stability in critical life choices such as values, interests, and friends. These critical life choices together contribute to a patient's self-concept: Who am I? What interests me? What are my beliefs? Identity consolidation is a critical variable because it so closely corresponds to an individual's sense of internal stability.

Object relations/interpersonal relations: During the course of the structural interview, the therapist will try to get a sense of the quality of important relationships in the patient's life. This line of questioning can include the patient's experience of prior treaters (Was the patient able to form a useful treatment alliance? How did the treatment end?), as well as co-workers, friends, and family. The therapist will be listening for the patient's capacity to form enduring relationships, with nuanced (vs. caricatured) experiences of others. The therapist will be interested in the patient's capacity for warmth and closeness and for the nature of the patient's expression of sexuality. Exploration of the patient's important relationships will give the therapist clues about the patient's internal object relations (mental representations of self in relation to others), as well as a preview of the patient's pattern of defensive functioning, as noted above.

Superego or moral values: The structural interview will explore areas of the patient's history and current functioning in a proactive way; the interviewer will probe any areas that seem confusing or contradictory, including aspects of the patient's life that might suggest compromised superego functioning. What are we referencing here? Any information suggesting a history of frank antisocial behavior – lying, cheating, or stealing – would be important areas to investigate. The patient's capacity for guilt, as well, would be a critical subject. At the other end of the spectrum, a system of excessively rigid values would reflect likely personality pathology. Why would a patient's moral values be relevant? They are crucial to a patient's self-acceptance and adaptive functioning within society. The TFP therapist will consider this subject when evaluating the patient's prognosis and when considering the relative stringency of the treatment frame.

Taken together, the TFP therapist's standard evaluation and enhanced exploration (informed by questioning and directly probing the RADIOS topics) enable the interviewer to speculate about the patient's "level of organization." This shorthand for a patient's capacity to function in critical areas lets the interviewer describe both the diagnostic category (or categories) in evidence and also more generally the patient's severity of illness. In the TFP nosology, the continuum extends from the most impaired patients (psychotic level of organization), through a broad category of patients in the borderline organization category (ranging from "lower borderline organization" including patients with borderline, schizotypal, antisocial, paranoid, schizoid, and hypochondriacal personality disorders, through "higher borderline personality organization" including patients with avoidant, dependent, histrionic, and sadomasochistic personality disorders), to "neurotic level of organization" including patients with obsessive-compulsive, depressive-masochistic, and hysterical personality disorders. Patients with narcissistic personality disorder can have highly variable presentations, ranging from those in the most severely impaired category, with near-psychotic organization, to lower, mid-, or even higher borderline organization, approaching a "neurotic" level of functioning.

As described, using the shorthand of level of organization allows the therapist to convey a lot of information in an economical way. When the therapist distills information and makes a guess about a patient's level of organization, this gives the therapist important information about risk, prognosis, probable response to treatment, and what treatments will most likely work, allowing the therapist to communicate in just a few phrases with colleagues about how impaired (or not) the therapist sees the patient.

1.4   Setting Goals

- *The TFP therapist enlists the patient to put into words specific personal goals, as well as treatment goals, as part of the evaluation process.*
- *Exploration of goals adds a dimension to the diagnostic assessment and fulfills the therapist's obligation to engage the patient in a discussion of informed consent.*
- *The TFP therapist keeps the patient's personal goals and treatment goals in mind, remaining vigilant to distractions from a focus on those goals as therapy proceeds.*
- *The process of having the patient articulate personal and treatment goals helps to avoid his or her chronically passive or apathetic participation.*

It is common for patients with significant personality disorder pathology to present for treatment feeling overwhelmed
or confused. Patients, understandably, may present their chief
complaints in ways that are inchoate or vague, often a challenge for the therapist who struggles to comprehend what the
patient wants and how the therapist can help. As mentioned
earlier, for some patients the experience of being in psychotherapy is a goal of its own, and the idea of using the psychotherapy to make changes outside of the treatment is a foreign
one. The TFP evaluation emphasizes discussion of a patient's
personal goals and treatment goals. These goals help orient
the therapist during the course of treatment and give the
patient and therapist a way to measure progress in the treatment over time. While this may seem obvious, clinical experience suggests that many patients with PD diagnoses engage in
extended, unguided treatments that reflect aspects of their
underlying psychopathology (e.g., an unconscious wish to be
cared for unconditionally by an ideal parental figure). When
the TFP therapist raises the issue of goals at the outset, the
therapist is communicating that this particular treatment is
designed for facilitating certain changes, and not one designed
for open-ended support and care.

The patient's response to questions about goals adds a
valuable dimension to the diagnostic assessment process.
Some of the areas highlighted in the previous sections –
defenses, object relations, identity consolidation vs. confusion – may be reflected in the patient's reaction to discussion
of goals. What are the differences between personal goals and
treatment goals? This question relates directly to the way
elucidation of goals is a critical part of the informed consent
process. The patient's personal goals pertain to the potential
changes in daily life – changes in work, studies, friendships, or
romance would be typical. Treatment goals may be less obvious; the assessment phase can lead directly into the possible
benefits and limitations of certain treatment interventions.
Take the example of the recent graduate who finds himself
fired from every new job, making it impossible to get traction
in his chosen field. His personal goal may be to stay employed

and figure out how to move up in the business world; a treatment goal may be to understand how his behavior impacts others, what may be happening in the workplace that alienates his employers but remains outside of his awareness. The informed consent process, as in any medical intervention, requires that the clinician and the patient together weigh risks and benefits; without a clear explication of the objective of the treatment, this process is not possible. TFP would not be the treatment of choice for the patient with the abstract goal of "self-discovery" or "learning to feel my feelings." There may be interventions for patients with those ambitions, but TFP would require more earthbound aspirations.

Also integral to the informed consent process is a discussion with patients about diagnosis. All the evidence-based treatments for BPD include explicit discussion of the borderline diagnosis as part of the intervention. There is not the same consensus about the value of sharing other DSM-5 personality disorder diagnoses with patients, even when reliably made. The rationale for discussion of the BPD diagnosis, or other PD diagnoses, even if done using the therapist's own nonclinical language, is multifaceted. Introducing discussion of the diagnosis can help patients in the following ways; stimulating the patient's interest in reflecting on his or her internal psychological world; giving patients a realistic appraisal of prognosis; helping guide patients to effective (evidence-based) treatments; empowering patients to learn about the disorder on their own, insuring patients are not subject to ineffective and potentially dangerous psychotherapeutic and pharmacologic interventions best suited to other disorders; and directing patients and families to identify useful advocacy groups that provide salient psychoeducation.

As we will see going forward, patients in a useful exploratory psychotherapy will grapple with painful matters; the TFP therapist will expect the patient, at times, to deflect attention from these matters to less freighted subjects. The TFP therapist will always keep in mind the principal goals of the treatment, alert to the risk of "trivialization" or the patient's tendency to engage in matters of limited consequence as a temporarily relieving but overall derailing coping strategy. The risk of trivialization is closely associated with a concerning passivity or apathy that can subtly creep into a treatment. The TFP focus on goals keeps the treatment from getting bogged down; it should be ever present and gently forceful.

1.5   Contracting and the Treatment Frame

- *The contracting phase follows directly from the assessment process; the therapist negotiates the treatment contract alert to elements of the patient's diagnosis and level of organization.*
- *The rigor of the treatment contract is directly related to the severity of the patient's disturbance.*
- *The treatment contract is designed to create a sense of reliability and safety for both the patient and therapist.*
- *The contracting process sets up the treatment frame; the therapist expects challenges to this frame that reflect aspects of the patient's internal world over time, to be examined together with the patient.*

Let's consider the challenges faced by clinicians hoping to engage BPD patients in treatment in the days before the development of evidence-based treatments, all of which as noted, include a focus on the treatment frame. In retrospect it stands to reason that the familiar symptoms of BPD – intense anger and distress, a pattern of unstable relationships, or transient psychosis in stressful situations – would make a productive engagement in treatment difficult and ruptures in treatment almost inevitable. With twenty-twenty hindsight, we now can see how a focus on the treatment frame would be critical in this population, in ways not fully appreciated in the past. In TFP, as in the other evidence-based treatments, attention to the treatment frame is understood as a critical means of patient retention. But in TFP, the focus on treatment contracting and the maintenance of the treatment frame is more than simply a tool for alliance and retention. The frame is the treatment's "canvas," and the therapist invests time and energy in establishing the treatment frame knowing that, inevitably, it will be challenged in ways critical to the *success* of the treatment.

This may seem counterintuitive; the therapist invests time and energy in the contracting process and in the maintenance of the treatment frame *expecting* challenges from the patient. Indeed the contracting phase follows the assessment process as the therapist is forewarned about possible pitfalls in the treatment informed by the tentative diagnoses made. In the treatment of the less severely impaired patient, the therapist may be generally conscientious about the treatment contract, but recognizing an increased severity of disturbance, the therapist is much more obligated to laboriously explore all the possible ways the treatment could be compromised. The therapist empathizes with the patient's periodic challenges or resistances to the treatment since the process of honest exploration of the full extent of the patient's internal emotional world inevitably touches on difficult and sometime painful topics and feeling states.

When we describe the treatment contract, it is natural to ask: Is it a written legal document? It isn't; the treatment contract is the oral agreement between patient and therapist. The contract covers basics universal to almost every psychotherapy process such as scheduling, cancelation policy, fees, and billing. In the treatment of patients with BPD or other more severe personality disorders, the contracting process must extend to detailed discussion of intersession contact, emergency policies, and hospitalization, among other topics.

Here is a list frequently cited contract elements:

- Scheduling process
- Starting and stopping sessions on time
- Patient hygiene
- Fees and payment schedule
- Cancelation policy
- A commitment to meaningful paid work, volunteer work, or studies
- Intersession contact
- Permission to contact family
- Permission to contact other treaters
- Adherence with medical care
- Adherence with laboratory testing
- Adherence with medication
- A requirement of abstinence from substance abuse, if indicated
- A plan for managing eating disorder symptoms, if indicated
- Participation in adjunctive treatments
- The patient's obligation to speak freely in sessions
- The patient's obligation to be honest
- Patient's threatening behavior
- Management of suicidal behavior
- Involvement of psychiatric emergency services
- Involvement of psychiatric inpatient services

Why all the fuss about a treatment contract? Why can't the treatment begin posthaste without a delay of days or even weeks spent reviewing details, contingencies, and consequences? Why not manage problems as they arise? On the surface, the PD patient presenting for treatment can appear to be the suffering, vulnerable party, asking for assistance from an empowered, skillful treater. As we will find, in the discussion of object relations dyad and their inverses, this dynamic will reliably be reversed. What would this reverse look like? Take the example of the BPD patient who presents as waif-like and disempowered, appealing to the "competent" therapist for a helping hand. Within weeks, in this story line, the therapist feels increasingly lacking in competence with every call from the patient threatening suicide; the waif-like patient has quickly become a powerful (albeit destructive) force, causing the therapist to feel deskilled and vulnerable. The treatment contract aims to protect the therapist, helping to create a safe and reliable treatment situation. Let's examine further the scenario introduced – the patient who becomes actively suicidal between sessions. In the classical DBT model, this patient could contact the therapist at will for phone coaching. In many treatments without a clear contracting process, the patient's suicidality between sessions would cause a crisis for the treater; the treater may have other patients scheduled, or other obligations, making availability to engage the suicidal patient between sessions impossible. The patient may find the contact with the therapist between sessions comforting or even exciting, leading, paradoxically, to an escalation of calls over time, even as the therapist offers intersession contact to help *contain* the patient's distress. In the TFP contracting process, the therapist will enlist the patient in a detailed discussion about intersession contact, underscoring the realistic limits to the therapist's availability and the use of emergency services as needed. This protects the therapist and reinforces for the patient the reality of the therapist's availability. Such a discussion can take effort; the patient may protest, family may see such a policy as depriving or even cruel, and a review of the many possible sequences of events can be time-consuming. The contracting process, in summary, tries to create a setting in which the patient is fully aware of his or her obligations and the consequences of his or her actions. At the same time the therapist should feel secure enough to be clear-thinking and attentive.

The creation of the treatment frame allows the therapist to learn about the patient through challenges to the frame that may be subtle or obvious. The therapist is always asking: What is the significance of the challenge to the frame and what does it mean about the patient's experience of the therapist? Many therapists grapple with the patient who comes late to sessions. During the TFP contracting phase, the therapist will convey the expectation that sessions begin and end on time; if it emerges that the patient, in a prior treatment, was not able to come to sessions in a timely manner, the therapist will want to know all the details. Because the patient and therapist had discussed timeliness during the contracting phase, once the treatment begins the patient's tardiness would be "fair game" for discussion. The therapist raising this issue would not do so in a punitive way; the therapist is genuinely curious, and the patient's lateness may be incidental, or it may be significant. The exploration of the patient's lateness will have more meaning *because the patient and therapist have a contract;* the patient's actions now have meaning in terms of their relationship, to be aired and understood.

The Applied Transference-Focused Psychotherapy Glossary

Affect Storm A patient's heightened affective state, often influenced by intense anger or paranoid thinking, necessitating a distinct type of response from the therapist.

Affective Dominance The content of a patient's material noted to have the most emotional resonance, considered a useful place for the therapist to focus, barring other considerations.

Borderline Personality *Organization* This term captures a group of patients including, but not limited to, patients with borderline personality disorder. Patients with borderline personality organization are distinguished by the nature of defenses employed (a significant contribution of splitting-based defenses), degree of identity consolidation (significant elements of identity diffusion), and capacity for reality testing (generally intact, although with the possibility of a transient loss of reality testing).

Clarification The therapist's request for additional details when anything the patient says is vague, confusing, or incomplete.

Confrontation The therapist's act of bringing to the patient's attention aspects of his or her communications that are somehow discrepant or contradictory.

Countertransference The therapist's experience of the patient, reflecting the realities of the patient's life, the specifics of the patient's presentation, elements of the therapist's own history, and what might be happening in the therapist's life.

Depressive Position A term used to convey a patient's ability to hold seemingly contradictory ideas simultaneously, allowing for a tempered, nuanced experience of self and others. This state is also marked by the patient's increased capacity for taking responsibility for aggressive behaviors and wishes.

Interpretation The therapist's hypothesis, offered to the patient as one possible way of understanding a particular conflict the patient has described, with the goal of making sense of aspects of the patient's experience or behavior that on the surface seems irrational or contradictory.

Levels of Organization This shorthand used in transference-focused psychotherapy conveys information about an individual's functioning informed by the therapist's observation of the patient's reality testing, aggression, object relations, identity consolidation, and moral values.

Malignant Narcissism The combination of narcissistic personality traits and the triad of some antisocial behavior, aggression experienced without marked conflict, and paranoia.

"Naming the Actors" The therapist's intervention of identifying the dominant dyad emerging in the material at hand and "naming" this dyad, including the patient's self-concept and experience of another and the affect associated with this experience.

Object Relations Dyad The patient's self-representation (how the patient experiences himself or herself), the object representation (how the patient experiences another), and an associated affect or feeling; a role reversal, or inversion of the dyad, can be identified when the patient assumes aspects previously ascribed to the other.

Paranoid Position The patient's overall experience of self and others when splitting-based defenses predominate, and the patient is susceptible to a pervasive sense of mistrust.

Repression-Based Defenses vs. Splitting-Based Defenses Defenses are universally employed psychological means to negotiate pressures of competing affects, drives, and external realities. **Repression-based defenses** (repression, isolation of affect, intellectualization, reaction formation) can confer more flexibility and are considered "mature," while **splitting-based defenses** (projection and projective identification, denial, alternating idealization and devaluation, omnipotent control) are more closely associated with personality rigidity and volatility.

Role Reversal An expectable pattern of behavior marked by a shift in the relationship between the patient and therapist. In the role reversal, the patient either (a) assumes certain characteristics (e.g., empowered or demanding) previously ascribed to the therapist, or (b) attributes to the therapist certain characteristics while simultaneously demonstrating these characteristics himself or herself

Secondary Gain of Illness The attention, support, or accommodations that might be provided for a symptomatic patient; secondary gain of illness may serve as a motivation, conscious or unconscious.

Structural Interview The specific, deliberate approach to patient evaluation used in transference-focused psychotherapy. The evaluation builds on the standard diagnostic assessment process but includes particular questioning techniques and lines of inquiry designed to shed light on both diagnostic categories and overall levels of functioning in multiple spheres.

Surface to Depth The therapist's general approach to exploring the patient's defenses beginning with those conflictual aspects of experience more available and less threatening to the patient, with a goal of deepening exploration as is tolerated.

Technical Neutrality The therapist's conscious attempt not to "side" with one particular aspect of the patient's makeup (e.g., prohibitive self-reproach, impulses to act on desires for pleasure) but rather to remain "neutral" in relation to competing forces within the patient in order to facilitate their exploration. The therapist strives for technical neutrality unless the patient's behavior merits "taking a side" for the patient's protection.

Three Channels of Communication Transference-focused psychotherapy's adjustment of standard psychoanalytic listening to privilege how the patient *acts* and how the therapist *feels*, as much, if not more, than what the patient says.

Transference The patient's total experience of the therapist reflecting aspects of the patient's makeup, personal history, and prior relationships, as well as various facts about the therapist.

Treatment Frame The agreement between clinician and patient explicitly outlining their respective responsibilities and the particular details of their professional relationship. This contract can include "nuts and bolts" concerns such as fee and cancelation policy, as well as details pertinent in the treatment of patients with personality disorders such as intersession availability and management of suicidality.

References

1. Clarkin JF, Foelsch PA, Levy KN, Hull JW, Delaney JC, Kernberg OF. The development of a psychodynamic treatment for patients with borderline personality disorder: a preliminary study of behavioral change. J Pers Disord. 2001;15:487–95.
2. Clarkin JF, Levy KN, Lenzenweger MF, Kernberg OF. The Personality Disorders Institute/Borderline Personality Disorder Research Foundation randomized control trial for borderline personality disorder: rationale, methods, and patient characteristics. J Pers Disord. 2004;18:52–72.
3. Clarkin JF, Levy KN, Lenzenweger MF, Kernberg OF. Evaluating three treatments for borderline personality disorder: a multiwave study. Am J Psychiatr. 2007;164:922–8.
4. Lieb K, Zanarini MC, Schmahl C, Linehan MM, Bohus M. Borderline personality disorder. Lancet. 2004;364(9432):453–61.

5. Sansone RA, Sansone LA. Borderline personality in the medical setting. Prim Care Companion CNS Disord. 2015. doi 10.4088/PCCC.14r01743
6. Sansone RA, Sansone LA. Borderline personality disorder in the medical setting: unmasking and managing the difficult patient. New York, NY: Nova; 2007.
7. Kernberg OF. Severe personality disorders: psychotherapeutic strategies. New Haven, CT: Yale University Press; 1984.
8. Kernberg OF. Structural interviewing. Psychiatr Clin. 1981;4:169–95.
9. Yeomans FE, Clarkin J, Kernberg OK. Transference-focused psychotherapy for borderline personality disorder: a clinical guide. Arlington, VA: American Psychiatric Publishing; 2015.
10. Lenzenweger MF. Epidemiology of personality disorders. Psychiatr Clin. 2008;31:395–403.
11. Grant BF, Chou SP, Goldstein RB, et al. Prevalence, correlates, disability, and comorbidity of DSM-IV borderline personality disorder: results from the Wave 2 National Epidemiologic Survey on Alcohol and Related conditions. J Clin Psychiatr. 2008;69(4):533–45.
12. Torgerson S, Kringlen E, Cramer V. The prevalence of personality disorders in a community sample. Arch Gen Psychiatr. 2001;58:590–6.
13. Widiger TA, Frances AJ. Epidemiology, diagnosis, and comorbidity of borderline personality disorder. In: Tasman A, Hales RE, Francis AJ, editors. Review of psychiatry. Washington, DC: American Psychiatric Press; 1989. p. 8–24.
14. Zimmerman MA, Mattia JI. Differences between clinical and research practices in diagnosis borderline personality disorder. Am J Psychiatr. 1999;156(10):1570–4.
15. Bender DS, Dolan RT, Skodol AE, Sanislow CA, Dyck IR, McGlashan TH, et al. Treatment utilization by patients with personality disorders. Am J Psychiatr. 2001;158(2):295–302.
16. Goodman M, Roiff T, Oakes AH, Paris J. Suicidal risk management in borderline personality disorder. Curr Psychiatr Rep. 2012;14(1):79–85.
17. Biskin RS, Paris J. Management of borderline personality disorder. Can Med Assoc J. 2012;184(7):1897–902.
18. Richter C, Steinacher B, Zum Eschenhoff A, Bermpohl F. Psychotherapy of borderline personality disorder: can the supply meet the demand? A German nationwide survey in DBT inpatient and day clinic treatment facilities. Community Ment Health J. 2016;52(2):212–5.

19. Gunderson JG, Links P. Handbook of good psychiatric management for borderline personality disorder. Washington, DC: American Psychiatric Publishing; 2014.
20. Weinberg I, Ronningstam E, Goldblatt MJ, Schecter M, Maltsberger JT. Common factors in empirically supported treatments of borderline personality disorder. Curr Psychiatr Rep. 2011;13(1):60–8.
21. Caligor E, Kernberg OF, Clarkin JF. Handbook of dynamic psychotherapy for higher level personality pathology. Washington, DC: American Psychiatric Publishing; 2007.
22. Normandin L, Ensink K, Kernberg OF. Transference-focused psychotherapy for borderline adolescents: a neurobiologically informed psychodynamic psychotherapy. Journal of Infant, Child and Adolscent Psychothearpy. 2015;14(1):98–110.

Chapter 2
Transference-Focused Psychotherapy (TFP) and Its Applications: The Initial Stage of Treatment, Interventions Repeated and Refined, and What Happens Over Time in the Therapy Model

1. *The therapist's challenges in the initial phase of TFP include: tolerating the confusion associated with severe PD pathology, "naming the actors" to orient the therapist and give the patient a sense of being understood, and managing affect storms.*
2. *The TFP therapist listens for material and observes interactions reflecting the dominant object relations dyads and begins to speculate about possible role reversals in evidence.*
3. *The TFP therapist uses the tools of clarification, confrontation, and interpretation in probing the areas of conflict, cued by the strongest feelings expressed by and/or those most accessible to the patient, with the aim of deepening exploration over time.*

(continued)

© Springer International Publishing Switzerland 2016   33
R.G. Hersh et al., *Fundamentals of Transference-Focused Psychotherapy*, DOI 10.1007/978-3-319-44091-0_2

(continued)

4. *The goals of TFP, which include the patient's increased capacity for self-reflection and an integration of positive and negative experiences of self and others, emerge with extended effort and progress that unfolds in a nonlinear way.*

2.1   Introduction

As outlined in Chap. 1, the TFP therapist approaches the process of an individual psychotherapy with a patient with significant PD pathology in a systematic, markedly deliberate manner. The therapist proceeds as follows: (1) the comprehensive diagnostic assessment, (2) discussion with patient about the therapist's diagnostic impression, (3) identification of the patient's personal goals and treatment goals, (4) an extended contracting phase, and (5) a meeting with the patient and important people in his or her life (spouse, parents, children), if indicated. (Chap. 4 on TFP and family involvement describes in detail the indications for such a meeting.) It is important to recall that such a precise set of interventions is *not* considered standard procedure in traditional psychoanalytic psychotherapies or psychoanalysis and differs significantly in content and process from the other evidence-based treatments for BPD.

This chapter will describe the way TFP as an individual psychotherapy unfolds after the initial phases of treatment – diagnostic assessment, discussion of diagnosis, elucidation of goals, and contracting – have been accomplished. This description will closely hew to the outline of the treatment as described in the TFP manual. That said, *the central hypothesis of "applied transference-focused psychotherapy" is that the component parts of TFP on their own can be useful to clinicians of all stripes and that employing elements of TFP can improve clinical care provided by therapists not necessarily wishing to or able to provide TFP as an extended individual psychotherapy.*

The assessment phase of TFP, anchored in use of the structural interview, will often, but not always, help the therapist accurately assess the patient's level of organization and therefore prepare the therapist for what is to come. While the therapist's accurate appraisal of the patient's diagnosis and overall functioning using the structural interview is optimal, the process is not foolproof; the therapist may diligently proceed through an extended assessment phase and arrive at a diagnosis and general appreciation of the patient's level of organization, only to be surprised by the material the patient introduces once the treatment begins. The point of an extended, even painstaking, assessment process is the possible, but not guaranteed, benefit it may give therapists – a way to calculate how the treatment may proceed and, in TFP parlance, how rigorous the treatment frame will need to be. Many trainees are introduced to psychotherapeutic approaches that are premised on a prospective patient's relatively high level of organization. Supportive psychotherapy approaches that might highlight the therapist's role as giver of advice, guidance, or reassurance may assume that the patient has a higher level of organization with routine use of more mature or adaptable defenses. The trainee therapist anticipating work with a "healthier" patient will undoubtedly be flummoxed when experiencing the fragmentation, chaos, and confusion often seen in patients with severe PD pathology. The therapist using the structural assessment process and expecting to work with a patient with a borderline organization, for example, will know to prepare for a treatment that will not unfold in an organized, steady, or easily understood way.

The TFP therapist beginning treatment with a patient with severe PD pathology will expect to experience some degree of confusion. The TFP approach encourages the therapist to surrender to this confusion, to soak it up, as it were, rather than reflexively move to organize the material presented by the patient. The TFP therapist will take this opportunity – surrendering to the confusion generated by the patient – to begin to speculate about the most evident object relations dyads in play. The therapist will use the three channels of communication to consider: "What is the patient saying about his/her experience of self and others and what is the associated affect?" The TFP therapist doesn't aim to organize the material presented by the patient, particularly if the material is largely inchoate, but the therapist does have the goal of listening for clues about the patient's self-concept, experience of others, and associated feelings, or affects. The therapist anticipating material presented in an easily comprehended manner from a patient with a higher level, neurotic organization might be moved to put in order the chaotic material described by the patient with severe PD pathology; this effort to "fill in the gaps" created by inconsistencies in the patient's presentation distances the therapist from the patient's internal experience. The TFP therapist has a goal only of putting into words the dominant object relations dyads emerging or "naming the actors," as if the therapist were observing a snippet of dramatic dialogue and direction.

The identification of the emerging dominant object relations dyad begins with the process of "naming the actors" but includes the therapist's speculation about ways the dyad as described or played by the patient may be turned on its head. This "role reversal" assumes that the patient and the other important figures are on a "two-way street" so to speak; the therapist begins to consider ways, at times, "the shoe may be on the other foot," and the attributes the patient may ascribe to others can, at times, be identified in the patient's own behavior, albeit outside the patient's full awareness.

Many psychotherapy trainees will voice a familiar refrain when in supervision: "What am I supposed to say to the patient?" The repertoire of interventions used repeatedly in TFP is central to any psychodynamic psychotherapy intervention – clarification of the patient's thoughts, confrontation of observed contradictions, and interpretations of underlying conflicts. Just as the structural interview is basically an intuitive process, so too these terms reflect the therapist's intuitive response to clinical material. Clarification, in this sense, means the therapist is asking, "Can you tell me more? Can you make this any clearer to me? Can you fill in the details?" Confrontation is the process of asking the patient to reflect on material that somehow seems contradictory or discrepant.

The therapist is asking "I notice you have said two things that seem at odds; have you noticed that too?" An interpretation is a hypothesis about the patient's motivation; the therapist is offering this as a guess, not making a pronouncement. The therapist is wondering aloud with the patient "Is it possible that you behave this way because of that feeling – that fear, that anxiety, that wish?" The therapist as observer is making a suggestion about the patient's motivation that may not necessarily be in the patient's awareness.

The TFP therapist will be faced with the decision of how and when to intervene as the patient follows the TFP agreement to speak freely. The TFP therapist will observe for what seems to be the most affectively dominant material, i.e., the material associated with the strongest feelings. As noted, the TFP therapist will be monitoring the three channels of communication in determining the affectively dominant material, aware that how the patient behaves or how the therapist feels may be as important in this determination as what the patient actually says.

What does the TFP therapist expect to happen over time? The therapist accepts two essential facts of the treatment: the therapist is required to juggle multiple foci of attention at once, and the therapist understands the treatment will progress in an uneven and unpredictable way. What are the "balls in the air" the therapist is juggling? As mentioned, attention to the treatment frame is paramount throughout the treatment, even when there is a well-defined treatment contract in place. In fact, the TFP therapist *expects* challenges to the treatment frame over time. The TFP therapist, as described, monitors three channels of communication continuously with emphasis on how the patient behaves and how the therapist feels. The TFP therapist actively assesses the dominant object relations paradigms as they emerge in the treatment, linking material the patient brings in from his/her life outside of treatment to the transference as it evolves in sessions. The TFP therapist will expect the initial transference to be one primarily informed by vigilance and mistrust or a "paranoid" transference. (A less common pattern would be an initial transference fully dominated by idealizing, positive feelings, presumably keeping at bay the more negative transference.) This should not suggest the frank paranoia of a primary psychotic disorder, but an attitude that grows out of primarily splitting-based defenses. This expectation of a primarily paranoid transference may be one of the most challenging (and counterintuitive) elements of TFP for novice therapists. The TFP therapist should not expect to be liked or admired or even respected by the patient; the TFP therapist aims to be courteous and curious and consistently *tolerant* of the patient's negativity or mistrust.

The TFP therapist keeps one eye on the patient's articulated goals at all times. The TFP therapist also aims to maintain a neutral stance – warm, interested, but not overtly opinionated unless the therapist feels such an intervention is warranted. What would warrant a departure from neutrality? Any behavior that would threaten the safety of the patient or that would seriously undermine the treatment process and could not be resolved by exploration, interpretations, and understanding.

How will the therapist and patient know if TFP treatment is working? The therapist will expect things to "heat up" in the treatment in the initial period of engagement as things "cool off" for the patient outside of treatment. This might mean the patient becomes more challenging or angry with the therapist as acts of impulsivity or destructiveness outside of therapy begin to diminish. The therapist will expect that the repeated use of clarification, confrontation, and interpretation will lead to a deepening of the material at hand. The patient's increased capacity for self-reflection and growing ability to stand back and observe the consequences of splitting-based defenses should follow. Over time, the therapist will expect improvements in the patient's life outside of treatment; TFP is not done "in a vacuum," and the therapist will repeatedly ask about the patient's work, friendships, or romance.

TFP theory borrows from the psychoanalyst Melanie Klein the terms of the paranoid and depressive positions [1]. These terms are a shorthand way of describing the patient's evolution in treatment. The paranoid position is understood as experience of self and others dominated by negativity and mistrust paired with a contradictory experience, often less in evidence, of a wish for ideal caring and unlimited accommodation. This position is rooted in the patient's fundamental denial of his/her aggressive emotions and projection of them on the surrounding world. This leaves the patient with a sense of seeking perfect goodness in a menacing world. The term "depressive position" describes an increased capacity for nuance, albeit associated with depressive affects resulting from two developments. The first is the loss of hope for a perfect caregiver (as well as a perfect self); this loss of hope/ belief in the naïve ideal other or self requires a phase of mourning before emotional stability can be achieved. The second cause of depressive affects is the remorse that results from the individual's shift to awareness that aggressive affects exist within the self and are not the monopoly of others. It may be confusing to think of the "depressive" position as the goal of treatment; it may be more useful to think of "depressive" in this case as a synonym for realistic and grounded or complex in contrast to simplistic. Furthermore, a complete treatment helps the patient move the sense of mourning and remorse of the depressive position to full acceptance of the complexity of the human condition.

2.2 The Initial Phase of TFP: Tolerating the Confusion, Naming the Actors, and Managing Affect Storms

- *The TFP therapist anticipates the initial confusion frequently encountered in the treatment of patients with severe PD symptoms.*
- *The process of "naming the actors" allows the therapist to describe to the patient the emerging dominant object relations dyads as a first step in the patient reflecting on them.*
- *The management of highly charged exchanges or "affects storms" requires the TFP therapist to focus on the patient's specific, intense experience of the treater.*

An understanding of the likely patterns of fragmentation and discontinuous affect states often observed in patients with severe personality disorder pathology will cue the therapist to expect a degree of confusion at the beginning of any treatment. What is meant by fragmentation? In this case we mean rapidly shifting experiences of self and of others, often associated with intense affect. The discontinuity in affect states over time closely correlates with the DSM-5 diagnostic criteria of mood reactivity in BPD. Let's look at two different patients who contact Ms. D., a social worker with a private practice, with the same chief complaint: "I may have depression."

Ms. A. is a 30-year-old nurse who describes a low-grade depression resulting from dissatisfaction in her work. Ms. A. feels she is not well treated by her supervisor, whom she previously admired, and believes she is unfairly faulted for errors at work that are not within her control. Ms. A. reports she is actively applying for other positions in the hospital but in the mean time has felt "low" with a diminished appetite, some difficulty falling asleep, and less than usual interest in being intimate with her fiancé. She tells Ms. D., the social worker, that she would prefer to avoid taking medication if possible, but worries that her mood disorder symptoms will compromise her ability to study for her upcoming master's degree exams.

Ms. B. is a 30-year-old nurse who describes a low-grade depression resulting from dissatisfaction in her work. Ms. B. feels she is not well treated by her supervisor, whom she previously admired, and notes her "depression" has increased since she threatened to punch her supervisor leading to her current probation. Ms. B. reports she has been distraught after this incident, particularly because she had long felt her supervisor to be a close ally and confidante. While Ms. B. suggests she may have symptoms of depressive disorder, she reports that an active sex life with her downstairs neighbor has been a notable source of pleasure while she has been off from work. Ms. B. says she is particularly disappointed in her internist who prescribed an antidepressant that she took "for one night – it almost killed me and I may have to sue him!"

A TFP therapist beginning treatment with Ms. B. might be tempted to organize the confusing material offered in the first sessions, but following TFP protocol would instead accept the inevitable confusion offered in the narrative and use the time to begin to consider the most prominent object relations dyads described. This would be in contrast to the therapist's attitude when meeting in the initial stages with Ms. A., who is able to lay out a coherent, cohesive story. Ms. A.'s cohesive story and understanding of the various strands of her life suggest an integrated identity and thus would situate her at a neurotic level of personality organization. When meeting with Ms. A., the therapist would ask questions to further organize the material offered; given Ms. A.'s higher level of personality organization, the therapist might feel comfortable offering a more clearly supportive treatment with an expectation that Ms. A. would be capable of using the therapist's suggestions and insights in a productive way. With Ms. B., the therapist would begin to consider the dominant dyad, say, dependent, needy childlike figure mistreated by a careless, callous adult. The therapist might respond to the kind of chaotic material offered by a patient like Ms. B. by "naming the actors" or putting into words elements of the scenarios of self and others.

The process of "naming the actors" has two goals: it should communicate to the patient a sense of being understood, and it should help the therapist orient him/herself in a sea of confusing clinical data. The intervention of "naming the actors" is offered to the patient as a guess; the patient may accept or reject the therapist's understanding. The therapist doesn't stand on ceremony but invites the patient to correct any errors. If Ms. D., the social worker, were to say to Ms. B. "You describe a situation with your boss and your internist as if you're a vulnerable child who is poorly cared for by an oblivious parent," then Ms. B. might accept or reject this hypothesis. Ms. B. might correct Ms. D. stating: "No, that's not it at all. It's like I'm abuse victim who suffers at the hands of a sadistic monster." As noted, the TFP therapist would not correct the patient but would continue to try to refine the emerging object relations dyad as additional clinical material is offered. In the case outlined, the therapist would continue to listen for similar episodes that might confirm this pattern as a recurrent experience of self and others referenced by Ms. B.

An especially challenging situation encountered by the TFP therapist often, but not always, in the early stages of treatment is the "affect storm." This expression aims to capture a patient's especially intense reaction to the therapist, often infused with paranoia or rage. The TFP therapist does not attempt to "talk the patient out" of an affect storm, does not try to reason with the patient, or to introduce leavening or distracting material. The management of the "affect storm" requires the therapist to use "therapist-centered interpretations." This concept, from the contemporary British psychoanalyst John Steiner, orients the exchange between patient and therapist in an affect storm to emphasize the patient's negative, often paranoid, feelings about the therapist [2]. If Ms. B. were to explode at Ms. D. during an early session, to accuse her of being just as callous or sadistic as her boss or her internist, Ms. D. might be tempted to respond defensively, saying "I'm only trying to get the full story from you!" If Ms. D. were to use a "therapist-centered interpretation" she might respond: "It's as if you see me as a cruel and hurtful authority figure, who really doesn't care about you at all." The goal of such an interpretation is not to change the patient's mind or make a case for the therapist's general good will but, rather, to contain the explosive affect and to assure the patient that the therapist, to some extent, can understand how the patient is experiencing the therapist at that moment. The therapist describes the patient's perception without denying it or confirming it; the ability to *consider* it can help the patient begin to reflect on, rather than simply react to such ideas.

2.3 Listening for the Dominant Object Relations Dyads as They Emerge and Speculating About Patterns of Role Reversal

- *The TFP therapist will begin to appreciate the dominant object relations dyads as they emerge in material from the patient's life and become evident in the transference.*
- *The TFP therapist will repeatedly articulate the most prominent dyads, refining description of the dyads in reaction to the patient's response.*
- *The TFP therapist will expect to identify patterns of role reversal within the dyads, meaning the patient behaving in specific ways that had routinely been ascribed to important others.*

As noted, the TFP therapist's initial response to the confusion often seen with patients with severe PD pathology is to tolerate the confusion and contain the impulse to make confusing material more logical. At the same time, the therapist will begin to pick out from the confusing material the emerging dominant dyads or the patterns of the patient's experience of him or herself and others in his or her orbit.

Let's return to Ms. B., the nurse on probation from her job. Ms. D., her therapist, begins to hear a familiar story involving Ms. B., often with a different cast of characters but the general pattern remaining consistent. In Ms. B.'s case, Ms. D. begins to hear material suggesting Ms. B. sees herself as unprotected and wanting and others in her world as callous and mean. Ms. D. also identifies a persistent affect state, in Ms. B.'s case feeling hurt and angry, in these situations. Ms. D. puts her observations into words and offers them to Ms. B., open to any disagreements or modifications Ms. B. might offer.

The TFP therapist listens closely for the emerging dominant object relations dyad in the material the patient brings into the session, but also begins to consider how such dyads might emerge in the relationship with the therapist. With Ms. B., for example, the therapist begins to see how some of the same elements evident in Ms. B.'s relationship with her supervisor and internist are perceptible in their developing relationship. This focus and speculation distinguish TFP from other treatments; this is the *focus on transference*, as advertised, based on the view that the transference is a direct window into the patient's internal world. How might Ms. D. introduce to Ms. B. the transference elements she observes in their interactions? Not in a presumptuous or authoritative way, to be sure. Not in a manner suggesting superiority or weighted down with jargon, either. The TFP therapist over time will weave into discussion of the patient's life outside of treatment pertinent observations about the patient's attitude toward and behavior with the therapist.

One key element of the TFP approach to treating patients with severe PD pathology that has been an area of controversy over the years is the TFP focus on the patient's aggression. This can be a confusing subject; what is meant by aggression, anyway – is it pushing into lines, getting into fights, or driving fast? Identifying aggression in this context is less obvious or concrete; it may be better understood as identification of an impulse to victimize others in those whose chief concerns or complaints relate to the experience of feeling victimized themselves. It should also be understood that aggressive affects are not, by definition, bad. Aggressive feelings, when successfully integrated into the personality, can be sources of ambition, competitiveness, and creativity.

As mentioned, Ms. B. recounts to her therapist in almost every session some variation on a theme of a vulnerable "victim" suffering at the hands of an irrational, cruel authority figure. Ms. B. began her treatment with such a story related to her supervisor at work; over time her therapist hears of other comparable scenarios – Ms. B. mistreated and maligned. As their treatment progresses, the therapist becomes aware of a growing sense of vulnerability *she* is feeling with Ms. B., as Ms. B. seems to find any number of faults in her therapist's behavior, often attacking her directly with caustic, taunting language. Here the patient exhibits behaviors she had previously ascribed to others and does so in a way that reflects such a pattern is outside of her awareness; this is the "role reversal" the therapist might expect in patients with severe PD symptoms.

As Ms. D., the therapist, becomes aware of this pattern of role reversal, she begins to compose a description of such behavior to propose to her patient Ms. B.

Ms. D. (therapist): "I've noticed since today's session began you've been raising your voice when describing the ways your sister is mistreating you; you seem particularly frustrated with me, feeling I'm not sensitive enough about the effects of her mistreatment."

Ms. B.: "You're just exasperating! I'm coming here for help; I'm telling you how my sister tortures me and you sit there with that ridiculous look on your face. You charge me money and end up siding with her, blaming me for everything."

Ms. D. (therapist): "You often tell me I act in the same way that your sister does, that I'm just as hurtful and abusive as she is, and we can look at that. However, I've been thinking about the nature of our communication here and what I'm about to say may come as a surprise. If you take a step back and look at the ways you've been acting toward me – raising your voice and dismissing my efforts – it's like the shoe is on the other foot, meaning your behavior toward me has some of the quality of mistreatment that you find in me with regard to you."

Here the therapist is attempting to bring to the patient's awareness aspects of her aggression not in the patient's awareness and likely to be a source of distress and dysfunction for her in her life outside of treatment. The therapist makes such a comment only after identifying the dominant dyad (in this case vulnerable patient victimized by cruel authority figure) and monitoring *her own* countertransference feeling of vulnerability, which inform her intervention.

2.4   How to Intervene: Identifying Affective Dominance and Repeatedly Using the Tools of Clarification, Confrontation, and Interpretation

- *The TFP therapist listens for the material associated with the strongest feelings expressed by the patient.*
- *The TFP therapist uses the tools of clarification, confrontation, and interpretation repeatedly over time.*
- *The therapist offers interpretations at a level of depth deemed most tolerable to the patient.*

Thus far, much of the description of TFP underscores the ways it fundamentally differs from traditional psychoanalytic psychotherapies. While this is definitely the case, TFP shares with psychoanalytic approaches the expectation that a patient will speak freely during sessions. The TFP contract reinforces this expectation; the therapist will not ordinarily direct the patient during their time together, although there are exceptions to this policy, as in any crises that might arise, or with direct threats to the treatment. The format of sessions will differ markedly from the standard medical or supportive psychotherapy model of the clinician determining the topic of conversation and asking the patient a series of related questions. For many, maybe most, patients, the expectation to speak freely and the absence of direction by the therapist is met with trepidation or laughter. "Am I just supposed to talk?" the patient may ask nervously. The TFP therapist may need to reinforce this expectation repeatedly and may need to reassure the patient that while it is common to find this process challenging, at least at the start, this method of participating in therapy helps gain access to deep levels of emotion and conflicts.

As the patient begins to speak freely, the therapist will try to determine the material offered by the patient that has the greatest affective intensity. Sometimes this may be obvious, easily determined by the content, by the patient's tone of voice, or by the patient's facial expressions. Sometimes determining the material of greatest affective intensity may be more challenging, particularly when there may be a discrepancy between an *absence* of expressiveness in evidence when the content of the material offered by the patient seems clearly fraught to the therapist. (For example, the patient who communicates in a dispassionate monotone, "Today is my twenty-fifth wedding anniversary." The therapist's observation about the patient's blunted affect when introducing this particular content would prompt the therapist to point out this discordance.) This process of identifying the material of affective dominance helps to orient the therapist; this should prompt the therapist to use the intuitive interventions of clarification and confrontation to bring critical aspects of the patient's internal world that might be shut out of awareness by dissociative defenses to light.

The presence of severe PD symptoms often has an impact on a patient's ability to share material in a coherent and easily understood way. Patients with BPD may demonstrate rapidly shifting experiences of self and others, making it almost impossible for the therapist to follow. Some patients with narcissistic traits may present material as if it were *assumed* that the therapist has the pertinent background information or knows the players involved in any particular story. The TFP therapist may spend much of the time in initial meetings asking for clarification of details. The therapist does so with genuine curiosity and thereby conveys to the patient a sincere interest in the details of the patient's life. The therapist will repeatedly intervene, asking "Can you tell me more? Can you be more specific?" The therapist will ask the patient to supply details to make clear any material that is vague or puzzling. There may be times when the patient will communicate that a particular subject is too difficult or distressing to explore; the TFP therapist will be respectful of the patient's wish to set limits on certain areas of exploration, but will remain curious about all subjects going forward, even those particularly sensitive or upsetting.

It should be apparent that the process of clarification, likely considered routine or benign in many clinical situations, could have considerable significance in the emerging transference in a TFP treatment. How might a relatively straightforward request for more information have such significance? A patient's lack of clarity may reflect shame or mistrust or dishonesty or the assumption that the therapist is omniscient and can understand without full explanation; the TFP therapist's request for more information may feel accusatory or intrusive with some patients. Alternatively, the patient with a more idealized experience of the therapist in the beginning of treatment may experience clarification questions as highly gratifying or even seductive. The point here is that consideration of transference and countertransference currents is part of TFP treatment from the very earliest stage of treatment. How and in what way the patient presents even the most basic material will have clinical significance.

The intervention of confrontation follows closely on the heels of clarification; confrontation will have particular resonance with severe PD patients because the process aims to bring into the patient's awareness aspects of his experience that are, at baseline, kept apart. Confrontation in this context has a different meaning than the more common definition that implies conflict or dispute; in this case, confrontation means the process of bringing to the patient's attention any information that might be at odds or discrepant. Again, the process of confrontation in TFP isn't a preamble to the treatment – it is *part* of the treatment, albeit in the guise of the therapist's data collection. Inquiring about a discrepancy in the patient's communication is an invitation for the patient to reflect. When the therapist points out to the patient, "You're saying now you feel this way about Maria; I'm struck because during our last meeting you said something very different about Maria," the therapist may be addressing aspects of the patient's splitting or alternating idealization and devaluation of another over time. The patient's reaction to such a confrontation may reflect a capacity for self-reflection, "I see that doesn't quite add up"; on the other hand, the patient could react with anger, responding: "I said that about Maria last time because she was so awful to me then; today I'm talking about how sweet she is. Can't you understand the difference?" Either response is useful information for the therapist; the latter response offers the therapist an opportunity to explore the patient's negative transference, considered essential in a TFP treatment.

Many novice therapists may feel a particular pressure to make "important" or "deep" interpretations, almost along the lines of now caricatured orthodox psychoanalytic pronouncements from another era. Often these novice therapists feel compelled to include in these interpretations material from the patient's distant past, as if the importance or depth of an interpretation requires it to include material from the patient's childhood. In TFP an interpretation is considered the therapist's hypothesis about the patient's motivation proffered only after an extended period of clarification and confrontation. The TFP therapist is always asking: If I offer the patient a hypothesis about his or her motivation, am I doing so in a way the patient can tolerate and use what I'm offering? This question reflects the overall stratagem of approaching the patient with a "surface-to-depth" appreciation of the patient's defenses. The defenses are there for a good reason; staying too long on the surface, the therapist might be focusing on material that is obvious or inconsequential; going too deep, the therapist might dismantle much-needed defenses, offering a hypothesis before the patient is ready to use it.

TFP interpretations will target distinct levels of the patient's functioning. These interpretations may include:

- The direct interpretation of particular primitive defenses and the ways certain maladaptive behaviors may help patients manage specific internal experiences
- The interpretation of the active object relations dyad and, if applicable, its reverse, as already described
- The interpretation of the way a particular object relations dyad, clearly evident on the surface, may keep at bay a contemporaneous object relations dyad that might be more anxiety producing for the patient

Let's return to Ms. B. and her therapist Ms. D. in discussion of these different subtypes of interpretation. Early in their work together, Ms. D. learns enough about Ms. B. and the particular primitive defenses she uses (and associated maladaptive behaviors) to feel confident enough to offer an interpretation to Ms. B. about specific internal experiences she speculates might be a particular source of distress to her. In Ms. B.'s case, one primitive defense identified might be splitting, or an alternating experience of another as either purely idealizing or devaluing, as in the case with Ms. B.'s supervisor at work. The associated maladaptive behavior in this case might be the acting out of threatening violence, a behavior with a variety of concerning repercussions. Ms. D. may interpret for Ms. B. that her growing attachment to her supervisor made her feel vulnerable in ways not fully in her awareness and that her intensely destructive outburst was a reaction to that vulnerability.

As outlined, the process of identifying a role reversal in an object relations dyad is a way the therapist can acknowledge a behavior split-off from the patient's awareness. The intervention of identifying such a role reversal in the patient's relationship with the therapist can be an unusually powerful and effective interpretation of this sort. In this case, the therapist is offering a hypothesis along the lines of: I'm wondering if the distress you describe as a steady barrage of ill will from others might, in fact, reflect a two-way street?

Over an extended period, when the TFP therapist has repeatedly focused with a patient on an object relations dyad on the surface, such as that observed in the case of Ms. B. and her therapist Ms. D., the therapist will begin to consider what defensive purpose it serves the patient to be mired in such a routine. It seems Ms. B., at least on the surface, can only operate on "two speeds," as it were; she is either feeling mistreated and rejected by others or, as her therapist points out, Ms. B. herself is mistreating and rejecting others with an equal, if not greater, vehemence. This possibility suggests one dyad, infused by paranoid thinking and negativity, may be a comfort of sorts in its own way. Ms. D. suggests this to Ms. B.:

"I'm wondering if being in a state of constant vigilance and mistrust, despite the toll it takes, confers some kind of comfort and reassurance for you. At least you know where you stand, as with your supervisor, your sister, or with me. I'm aware that despite your stated displeasure with me and with our work together, you nevertheless come to every session. This suggests to me you have some good feelings for me, maybe even a growing dependence, and that these positive feelings are threatening in their own way. If you have positive feelings for me you're *really* vulnerable; you just don't know what I might do to you in that case."

An interpretation like the one above is done only after considerable preparation; the therapist wants to know if the patient can tolerate such an exchange and wants to have some optimism such a hypothesis if offered might be useful to the patient; this is the "surface-to-depth" concept. The therapist may have had an inkling for some time about the way the object relations dyad on the surface helped the patient manage anxieties associated with the object relations dyad kept outside of her awareness; following the TFP approach, the therapist would have waited patiently until she had confidence the patient could hear and use such an observation.

2.5   What Happens Over Time: Increased Self-Reflection, Integration of Positive and Negative Feelings, and Improved Functioning Outside of Treatment

- *The overarching goals of an individual TFP treatment are the modulation and integration of extreme positive and negative experiences of self and others: the integration of identity.*
- *The patient's increased capacity for self-reflection should follow the deepening of treatment over time.*

(continued)

(continued)

- *The TFP therapist will expect positive changes in the patient's life outside of treatment.*
- *The TFP therapist will monitor for evidence of the evolving depressive position as it replaces the generally dominant paranoid position over time.*
- *While TFP has a specific trajectory for an individual treatment, the component parts of TFP have value on their own.*

TFP as an individual treatment has a defined trajectory; the TFP therapist has a number of aspirations for the treatment, a combination of personality changes (perhaps more simply described as the patient's improved coping strategies and an appreciation of the depth and complexity of self and others) and actual changes in aspects of the patient's life outside of the treatment. TFP is not, by any means, a brief treatment intervention; the TFP therapist will estimate the duration of the treatment to be somewhere between 1 and 3 years, sometimes more. Obviously such an extended treatment might not fit well when a "quick fix" is expected. Regardless of the duration of the treatment, an "applied TFP" philosophy would identify potential gains for the patient at every step of the treatment, even if it were not to unfold in a "platonic" or ideal way.

When Ms. D., the social worker, first encountered Ms. B., the nurse on probation from her job following a threat to harm her supervisor, Ms. D. immediately sensed she would need to proceed with TFP "by the book" given the acuity of the case and her own countertransferential anxiety. Ms. D. proceeded stepwise with the many required elements of the treatment including:

1. Assessment using the structural interview.
2. Generation of a differential diagnosis including standard DSM-5 nosologic categories, as well as specific personality disorder traits and diagnoses.
3. Explicit discussion with the patient about the personality disorder diagnosis made and the ways its course and treatment would differ from a primary mood disorder presentation. (Recall Ms. B.'s chief complaint that she believed she might be suffering from "depression.")
4. An extended contracting phase with ample opportunity to air Ms. B.'s objections to elements of the treatment frame as outlined by Ms. D. Given Ms. B.'s history of a threat of violence toward her supervisor, Ms. B. stressed the treatment-threatening potential of similar behavior going forward.
5. An explicit discussion of Ms. B.'s personal goals and treatment goals.
6. Ms. B.'s consent for Ms. D. to review the case with Ms. B.'s prescribing internist.
7. A meeting with Ms. B.'s sister, her closest family member, to review the diagnosis, details of the treatment, and risks and benefits of alternative treatment interventions.

Ms. D. began her work with Ms. B. aware of the multiple elements of the treatment that she would be required to monitor as the treatment unfolded. These elements included:

1. Orientation to Ms. B.'s personal goals (returning to her work as a nurse and developing a career, finding a relationship that would allow her to combine passion and companionship) and treatment goals (understanding her pattern of self-defeating behavior and difficulty combining closeness and sexual satisfaction)

(continued)

(continued)

2. Ms. D.'s attunement to the three channels of communication
3. Identification of the affectively dominant material during each session
4. Continued attention to the treatment frame and exploration of challenges to the frame as they arise
5. Continued refinement of Ms. D.'s identification of the dominant object relations dyads in evidence and consideration of role reversals
6. Use of clarification, confrontation, and (eventually) interpretation to expand the material offered by the patient and to engage the patient by offering speculation about unconscious processes
7. Ms. D.'s priority of maintaining a neutral stance, unless some aspect of Ms. B.'s behavior (e.g., a threat to physically harm someone) required deviation from this neutrality
8. Speculation about contemporaneous dyads and the interplay between dyads, more specifically, the ways a dyad on the surface might be shrouding a coexisting dyad, which might somehow be more threatening or less tolerable

As will be outlined in the coming chapters, clinicians may apply these individual elements in varying clinical situations. Clearly some of the TFP interventions are likely only useful when applied during the course of an extended individual psychotherapy, while others will have more broad utility.

What are Ms. D.'s overarching goals for her treatment with Ms. B.? How will she know if TFP is working as a treatment? As noted, Ms. D. expected the treatment to "heat up" in the initial stages as things "cooled off" in Ms. B.'s life outside of treatment. In the early stages of treatment, Ms. D. received concerned phone calls from Ms. B.'s sister; over time she stopped receiving those calls. Ms. B. followed the contract she and Ms. D. established and returned to her job part-time. As Ms. D. anticipated, the early months of the treatment were marked by repeated exploration of Ms. B.'s paranoid transference toward Ms. D.; Ms. B. came to their sessions, but she repeatedly questioned Ms. D.'s motives and faulted her for what Ms. B. perceived to be "errors" in her approach. Ms. D., rather than shying away from Ms. B.'s criticism and suspicion, mined Ms. B.'s complaints for additional information.

Ms. B.'s treatment proceeded with a typical "saw tooth" pattern. She would make some improvements in her outside life (she returned to work, she started dating) and seem to settle into the treatment, only to miss a number of appointments or challenge some other aspect of the treatment contract. Again, Ms. D. made such behaviors the focal point of their sessions; she repeatedly and consistently conveyed to Ms. B. in her actions that she could tolerate her negative feelings and aggression as long as they continued in their work with a sturdy frame intact.

Ms. D. began to observe in Ms. B. the gradual development of a more self-reflective perspective. The repeated use of clarification and confrontation contributed to this process; Ms. D. would consistently ask to learn more from Ms. B. and would bring to Ms. B.'s attention material that seemed somehow contradictory to her therapist. Ms. D.'s interpretation of the role reversals she witnessed, while at first a source of surprise and protest from Ms. B., appeared to take hold and lead Ms. B. to a pattern of increased self-awareness. Ms. B.'s increasingly regular attendance and growing capacity to speak freely about important and difficult subjects suggested to Ms. D. that despite her continued superficial antagonism toward her therapist, she was, in fact, growing more comfortable and even dependent. Ms. D. offered this observation to Ms. B. only after many months of treatment and only as Ms. B. continued to consolidate the gains she was making outside of treatment.

As described, the TFP therapist will actively monitor the critical elements of the patient's life outside of treatment. While it is true that the patient is expected to speak freely at each session, the TFP therapist will initiate discussion of topics critical to the patient's functioning outside of treatment if the patient does not spontaneously raise such matters. In the clinical material supplied above, for example, Ms. D. would routinely ask Ms. B. about her work performance or her dating life, if material related to these topics was not initiated by Ms. B.

The TFP therapist expects that much of the work done with patients with severe PD pathology in the early and midphases of treatment will be marked by a predominantly paranoid transference. This particular observation may seem misguided, if not downright mistaken, by many clinicians unfamiliar with TFP. Very often clinicians who engage with patients in an extended, supportive treatment dominated by the patient's superficial idealization of the therapist will find the idea that a paranoid transference – wariness with regard to the therapist – should predominate to be absurd. This is the familiar scenario of the therapist who feels he/she has a "good" relationship with the patient, who has endeavored to "work hard" on the patient's behalf over an extended period, only to find the treatment is not progressing and that the patient's aggression (e.g., a wish to defeat or humiliate the treater) has been driven underground (such a clinical situation is included in an article on the use of TFP concepts in consultations for *Overwhelming Patients and Overwhelmed Therapists*) [3]. Extended work in the paranoid transference is the expectable part of work with patients in what Melanie Klein called the "paranoid position [4]." As TFP treatment progresses, the therapist begins to notice elements of the "depressive position" that while not wholly dominating, become more apparent. The therapist will begin to appreciate the patient's more integrated and nuanced experience of self and others. Harsh, caricatured, or one-dimensional appraisals are softened; the patient is increasingly able to hold on to positive experiences of self and others, even in more stressful situations. It is, of course, somewhat counterintuitive to suggest that a "depressive" state would be the result of a helpful treatment. In Ms. D.'s treatment of Ms. B., the therapist recognized aspects of the emerging depressive position as Ms. B.

came to terms with the loss of the previously held wish for an experience of an ideal boss or boyfriend. The loss of the transiently intoxicating "all good" or "all bad" experiences is only partially cushioned by Ms. B.'s new stability. Ms. B.'s wistful recall of that old order suggests to her therapist the emergence of a kind of "depressive" state, while as a result of their work together, Ms. B. is showing evidence of an increased capacity for integration of feelings; it comes with the loss of a hoped for ideal but with a much-improved relationship with reality.

References

1. Klein M. Notes on some schizoid mechanisms. Int J Psychoanal. 1946;27:99–110.
2. Steiner J. Psychic retreats: pathological organization of the personality in psychotic neurotic and borderline patients. London: Routledge and the Institute of Psychoanalysis; 1993.
3. Carsky M, Yeomans FE. Overwhelming patients and overwhelmed therapists. Psychodyn Psychiatry. 2012;40(1):75–90.
4. Klein M. Envy and gratitude, a study of unconscious sources. New York: Basic Books; 1957.

Chapter 3
Transference-Focused Psychotherapy (TFP) Principles in Clinical Crisis Management

1. *Crisis management can be among the most challenging aspects of treating patients with personality disorders (PDs) and may engender the aversion to treating this population some clinicians experience.*
2. *TFP principles can give clinicians knowledge, attitudes, and skills useful in managing patients in crisis in varied settings.*
3. *TFP was developed as an individual psychotherapy for borderline personality disorder (BPD), but its theory and approach are of use in patient crisis management in other settings.*
4. *The TFP contract (in psychotherapy) has contingencies for expectable crises.*
5. *Clinicians interfacing with PD patients in crisis (in routine outpatient care, day treatment or intensive outpatient programs, medical settings, emergency rooms, or inpatient psychiatric units) will need to assess for transition to higher levels of care.*
6. *TFP principles add a dimension to the basic risk management tools used in treating PD patients in crisis.*

© Springer International Publishing Switzerland 2016 59
R.G. Hersh et al., *Fundamentals of Transference-Focused Psychotherapy*, DOI 10.1007/978-3-319-44091-0_3

3.1   Introduction

TFP was developed initially as an individual psychotherapy for patients with borderline personality disorder (BPD). The theoretical foundations of TFP, informed by psychoanalytic object relations theory, stress the borderline personality organization (BPO) patient's predominant use of *splitting-based defenses*, distinct from *repression-based defenses*, more often used by patients with neurotic personality organization (NPO). The splitting-based defenses are understood as key elements contributing to the symptoms experienced by BPO patients – including crises – and observed by clinicians attempting to help them.

TFP as an individual therapy stresses the need for an extended contracting phase with development and maintenance of the treatment frame over the course of the psychotherapy. The frame is understood as essential in allowing the BPO patient's pathology to unfold in a safe and secure setting and in facilitating joint exploration of the patient's internal world by the patient and therapist. The TFP contracting phase anticipates crises of varying kinds, according to the patient's specific clinical presentation, and compels the therapist and patient to develop a plan *in advance* of these crises. The TFP clinician appreciative of BPO and its associated compromised coping styles will anticipate future crises even in cases without histories of significant past personal or clinical crises. The contracting phase focuses on the patient's past experiences, including prior treatments, to predict challenges to the treatment frame in the future. The contracting phase explores issues such as non-adherence of different kinds, any behaviors likely to interfere with the effectiveness of the psychotherapy (substance use, eating disorders, recurrent suicidality), and neglect in attending to the realities of the patient's life outside of treatment. This process at once anticipates and aims to limit treatment-interfering activities often, but not always, presenting as personal crises for patients.

While the contract and treatment frame generally lead to a decrease in patients' acting out behaviors, clinicians engaged in TFP with BPO patients will expect some, though not all, patients to have crises of varying kinds during the course of treatment. This expectation informs first the evaluation process, then the contracting phase, and finally the ongoing maintenance of the frame throughout the treatment. TFP-trained clinicians are prepared for clinical crises from the outset and have the treatment contract and the needed predictability of the treatment frame for their support.

Many clinicians understandably find managing crises of BPO and BPD patients vexing, explaining in part the widespread aversion many clinicians feel about treating these patients [1, 2]. BPD patients are often seen by clinicians in crises of different kinds. In fact, BPD patients are *known* for their pattern of crisis-driven behavior, including affective instability, unstable relationships, suicide attempts and gestures, impulsivity in multiple spheres, and heightened response to real or imagined abandonment [3]. The splitting-based defenses believed to contribute to these behaviors include: splitting, projection and projective identification, primitive idealization and devaluation, denial, and omnipotent control. These defense mechanisms can distort understanding and interactions. Clinicians who do not have an appreciation of these mental mechanisms, and a coherent overarching approach to them, may understandably feel fearful, deskilled, or angry when assuming responsibility for patient care in situations as described.

TFP training can be of use to clinicians in crisis management of BPO and BPD patients even if those clinicians do not provide patients with extended individual psychotherapy [4]. TFP theory provides clinicians with a way to think about patients in the evaluation and diagnostic phase of treatment that will alert them to crises likely to emerge during the course of different treatments. TFP training can help clinicians develop attitudes that can aid them during affectively charged episodes with patients. The skills used by TFP therapists can be adapted by clinicians for use in crisis management in settings distinctly different from an extended, individual psychotherapy.

Psychiatrists, psychologists, nurse practitioners, social workers, and internists, among others, routinely interface with patients with personality disorder symptoms throughout the healthcare system. Medical professionals of all stripes are on record as wanting guidance about optimal treatment of the patient with PD symptoms in these settings, particularly the patient in crisis [5, 6]. Currently the fallback approach for many clinicians is generic support and validation often combined with hasty use of benzodiazepines or antipsychotic medications.

Education and training about personality disorders are virtually nonexistent outside of mental health settings. Even within mental health training programs, time devoted to education about personality disorder diagnoses is limited, which is regrettable given high rates of PD diagnoses in many outpatient and inpatient settings [7]. Clinical experience suggests that even now many clinicians are either unfamiliar with personality disorders or, if familiar, reluctant to make a personality disorder diagnosis [8]. Research indicates that even clinicians in well-established academic mental health settings may be likely to avoid exploring with patients aspects of their chief complaints or histories that might yield a reliably made personality disorder diagnosis [9]. The upshot is a population of PD patients with relatively high morbidity and mortality who may not be aware of their diagnoses and a wide range of clinicians who may find themselves treating PD patients in crisis who do so without the benefit of confidence in their diagnostic impression to guide their interventions.

A common scenario across healthcare settings: the clinician who initiates treatment with a patient unaware of a primary or co-occurring personality disorder. At some point in the treatment, the PD symptoms emerge and become the central focus of the clinician-patient relationship, often in a crisis situation. The clinician can become drawn into a maelstrom of confusion, unable to provide help to the patient in his or her routine, reliable way. The clinician may be aware of unusual feelings (guilt, anger, resignation), while the patient responds to the treater's interventions in unexpected and confusing ways.

Clinicians are often faced with the challenge of determining the optimal level of care for PD patients in crisis. Recurrent, disruptive, ineffective, and expensive psychiatric hospitalizations are often cited as a common pitfall in treating patients with BPD [10]. TFP principles can add a dimension to the complicated process of risk/benefit assessment for changes in levels of care.

While clinicians may be able to manage some PD patients in crisis with standard skills and interventions, the particular dynamics of certain personality disorders can create unusually complicated and sometimes dangerous situations. TFP training may add a useful dimension to standard risk management strategies. The risk management literature underscores specific elements of certain personality disorder presentations likely to increase a clinician's vulnerability [11]. It is easy to imagine the risks which can emerge for the clinician managing the PD patient in crisis; these can include deviation from standard practices, boundary violations, and unusual medication recommendations.

3.2   TFP Principles for Crisis Management Applied Across Treatment Settings

- *TFP, originally developed as an extended individual psychotherapy for BPD, has principles useful in the management of patients with PD symptoms in crisis in other settings.*
- *TFP-informed crisis management is based on an object relations theory of personality disorder symptoms.*
- *TFP-informed crisis management stresses understanding of the BPO patient's splitting-based defenses.*
- *TFP-informed crisis management stresses particular attention to the clinician's countertransference and the patient's nonverbal communication.*

The influence of psychoanalytic theory has waned considerably in recent years in many health professional training programs. Clinicians trained in the recent years, including psychologists and psychiatrists, may have only a limited familiarity with psychoanalytic concepts including object relations theory. It may therefore be surprising to suggest that a psychoanalytically informed approach to patients in varied settings could be of use to busy clinicians in a "real-world" setting today.

TFP was developed to treat patients with BPD, patients who generally had *not* responded to traditional psychoanalytic psychotherapy or state-of-the-art pharmacotherapy. This approach was directly and explicitly informed by these patients' histories of treatment failures marked by difficulties making and maintaining a treatment alliance, clinicians' aversion to working with patients prone to anger and suicidality, and the sorry reality of multiple iatrogenic complications seen in work with this population including recurrent, disruptive hospitalizations and harmful and ineffective polypharmacy.

TFP's design as an extended individual psychotherapy anticipates patients' crises, understood as a reflection of splitting-based defenses, which can undermine the patients' functioning in key spheres in their lives. Use of these more "primitive" or splitting-based defenses threatens certain patients' ability to benefit from psychotherapy in ways not seen with patients operating on a more highly functional or "neurotic" level.

The clinician versed in TFP principles derived from individual psychotherapy treatment can easily apply those principles in other settings. Common sense suggests that PD patients will be found throughout the healthcare system (and elsewhere including colleges and universities, the armed forces, and the criminal justice system). Unfortunately, lack of understanding about PDs and an unfortunate consensus that PD symptoms are to be treated only in specifically designed, extended psychotherapies have not helped those clinicians seeking guidance, particularly in crisis management.

TFP departs from traditional psychoanalytic psychotherapy practice in a number of fundamental ways. One overarching distinction is the TFP therapist's prioritizing of the three channels of communication. Traditional psychoanalytic psychotherapy privileges *what the patients says*, while TFP tends to focus on *how the patient behaves* and *the therapist's own reactions to the patient.*

Dr. P. Uses TFP Techniques She Learned as a Resident to Manage a Patient on a Medical Service

Clinical vignette: During her psychiatry residency, Dr. P. participated in a set of courses teaching the application of TFP principles. Dr. P.'s training began with a series of five lectures about the structural interview, a method of diagnostic assessment that moves beyond the standard descriptive psychiatry assessments done at her various training sites. Dr. P. also had lectures on TFP and its similarities to and differences from the other evidence-based interventions for BPD. A 1-year senior seminar on "applied TFP" allowed Dr. P. to review in a classroom setting recorded sessions of her work with a Veterans Administration patient with a history of recurrent suicidality and disruptive affective instability.

Dr. P. began a fellowship in consultation-liaison psychiatry with a specialization working with oncology patients. Early in her fellowship she was called to the medical floor for an "emergency" consultation. She was warned that the patient involved, while not particularly ill, had been disruptive with the nursing and medical staff and was acting both "paranoid and accusatory" in the context of her imminent discharge.

Before she had arrived on the floor, Dr. P. was aware of her own countertransference (apprehension) and her suspicion that the patient's presentation might reflect elements of a PD diagnosis exacerbated by a serious, but not life-threatening, medical illness. Dr. P.'s review of the patient's chart suggested a pattern of affective instability during her prior hospitalizations, not frank psychosis, marked by hostility and mistrust. Dr. P.'s initial meeting with this patient reinforced her consideration of a particular object relations dyad in play; in this case, the vulnerable and powerless patient enraged with what she felt was an indifferent and punitive medical staff. Dr. P. also took note of the cowering student nurse who had borne the brunt of this patient's verbal abuse, an observation that did not, at first, correspond to the dyad that Dr. P. was considering.

(continued)

(continued)

Dr. P. reviewed the notes from the medical attending who wondered if the patient in question might be "manic" given her pressured speech and irritability. Dr. P.'s interview was more consistent with PD symptoms and, in her mind, a dyad of threatened patient and abusive medical staff in which the roles could reverse to threatening patient and powerless staff. Dr. P. saw her role in the consultation as attempting to make an empathic connection with the patient by "naming the actors" (articulating the likely activated dyad, with a goal of containment) and inviting the patient to consider a projection by asking her to "see both sides" (identifying the dyad as the patient viewed and experienced it, and proposing consideration of its inverse, which up to that point had been out of the patient's awareness).

Dr. P. engaged the patient by first describing the observable dyad (threatened patient/hostile staff) and then suggesting its inverse (threatening patient/cowering staff) was also in play. The patient's response was a partial but helpful reduction in disruptive behavior. Dr. P. was able to defuse the situation without resorting to special arrangements of any kind or use of tranquilizing medication.

Take Home Point: Clinicians can use elements of TFP in clinical situations other than an extended individual psychotherapy.

3.3 Contingencies for Expectable Crises in the TFP Contract for Psychotherapy

- *The TFP contracting phase explicitly anticipates possible crises in the treatment.*
- *The ongoing maintenance of the treatment frame in TFP confers a degree of safety and security for the patient and therapist given the probability of disruptive crises.*

(continued)

(continued)

- *The TFP therapist establishes parameters related to treatment-threatening behaviors including eating disorders, substance use, and suicide gestures and attempts.*
- *The TFP therapist will depart from a technically neutral stance in certain crises with the goal of returning to this stance after a crisis is resolved.*

The TFP contracting phase follows the evaluation process anchored by the structural interview. The clinician identifying PD symptoms, particularly mid- or lower-level BPO, will therefore pay particular attention to the contracting phase given an understanding of BPO defensive operations. While this principle originated in the setting of long-term individual psychotherapy, it can be helpful in other treatment settings [12].

Clinicians often begin psychotherapy treatments without either a rigorous diagnostic assessment process or an extended contracting phase. This may be a reasonable approach for certain neurotic patients, but clinical experience suggests doing so with most BPO patients may set up the treatment for future derailing disruptions. The TFP approach *assumes* future crises and plans accordingly. In fact, a psychotherapy without crises of some kind would be seen by a TFP therapist as persistently and unhelpfully superficial given the nature of borderline organization. The absence of any crises would suggest that important parts of the patient's internal experience were being split off and kept out of the treatment setting. The expectation is that predictable crises will develop from the patient's splitting-based defenses and associated oscillations in the dominant object relations paradigms.

The TFP therapist makes a point of openly discussing likely future crises at the outset of treatment. This approach is distinctly different from that of the clinician who fears raising the issue of future crises as though discussing them would make them more likely to occur. (What if the patient has a substance use relapse? What if the patient becomes suicidal again?) The

TFP approach directly confronts an unspoken concern that exploring likely future crises might "plant an idea" in the head of a suggestible patient. In fact, the therapist's willingness to discuss possible crises may reassure the patient about the therapist's confidence in dealing with them.

In the TFP contracting phase, the clinician will painstakingly consider all the possible crises which might occur and therefore threaten the psychotherapy. The clinician will take each set of risks (substance use, eating disorders, non-adherence with medication, self-destructive behavior, etc.) and actively engage the patient in a prospective exploration of these possibilities. The clinician engages the patient in the contracting process so that it will serve as a touchstone for them both going forward.

Suicidal acts, threats of suicide, or non-suicidal self-injurious behavior are the crises most often associated with BPD [13]. Suicidal behavior is often seen in patients with other PDs as well including dependent, narcissistic, and antisocial personality disorders, although with different and distinct patterns in each case. Anticipation of suicidal thoughts or behaviors requires extensive discussion in the TFP contracting phase of the therapist's and patient's roles in managing these events. The TFP therapist accepts the high probability that suicidality and its meanings will be critical topics to be explored in the psychotherapy but consciously distinguishes between the services offered by the therapist (regular outpatient meetings with the goal of exploring the deepest levels of the patient's affects and conflicts) and those available to the patient in crisis in settings better suited to crisis management involving suicidality (emergency rooms, observation beds, inpatient psychiatric units). In the contracting phase the therapist treating the suicidal patient aims to accomplish two goals: first, create a treatment environment so that the therapist feels safe enough to provide effective treatment, and second, clarify his/her role and the nature of the therapy, which can include confronting the patient's expectation that the therapist might be available at all times to assist in crisis management. The position of TFP is that offering the patient "around the clock" access to the therapist would support the BPO patient's unrealistic longing for a "perfect provider" and that it would not support the patient's progress toward increased autonomy.

The TFP therapist makes great efforts to maintain a stance of technical neutrality. This approach differs from the supportive psychotherapist's comfort with "taking sides" and making explicit recommendations – something done in TFP only in rare situations when the patient presents an acute risk of self-destructive behaviors and does not respond to the therapist's attempts to address this risk with understanding and interpretation. The therapist's goal of maintaining technical neutrality will often be challenged during patient crises. Clinicians frequently find themselves defensive or critical with patients during crises; the TFP approach supports the goal of returning to a "neutral stance" following crises with an expectation of eventual exploration with the patient of the factors contributing to the crisis once the patient's safety is affirmed.

Ms. R. Provokes Her Therapist by Showing Evidence of Ms. R.'s Repeated Self-Injury

Clinical vignette: Ms. R. was discharged after a brief hospitalization following an episode of self-injury by cutting her antecubital fossa with an x-acto knife following an argument with her parents. Ms. R. had previously been in a supportive psychotherapy during a period of 2 years when she had repeatedly cut herself in this way, leading to one extended stay in a partial hospital program and one previous, brief hospitalization when she was evaluated at a community hospital emergency room and deemed "suicidal" even though Ms. R. reported she never had urges to end her life.

With her previous therapist, Ms. R. developed a pattern of showing her therapist the healing scars at each session. This became challenging for the therapist who felt unsure about how serious these wounds were and pressured to assume a role she felt would be better served by an internist. Ms. R.'s new therapist became aware of this pattern during the assessment phase and conveyed to Ms. R. during

(continued)

(continued)

the contracting phase that she expected such crises would likely occur going forward and that they were obliged to put a plan in place to manage these expectable crises. Ms. R.'s new therapist explained that the treatment plan would include the understanding that Ms. R. go to her internist to have her wounds evaluated with every cutting episode and that they would not meet in psychotherapy after a cutting episode until this occurred.

Ms. R. protested that she did not expect she would cut herself again but agreed to this arrangement. Two months later Ms. R. cut herself deeply after a falling-out with a friend. She came to her psychotherapy session and asked her therapist to look at her wound, which she reported was painful. The therapist reminded Ms. R. of their contract and ended the session with the plan to meet with Ms. R. again after hearing from her internist who had examined the wounds.

Take Home Point: The therapist can use the TFP contracting intervention to set limits on provocative behavior and insure that the treatment environment is comfortable for the patient and the clinician.

3.4   The Challenges of Managing Crises and Clinicians' Aversion to Treating Patients with Personality Disorder Diagnoses

- *PD pathology can add an element of urgency to any clinical situation.*
- *Clinicians may avoid exploration of PD symptoms and may be reluctant to make a personality disorder diagnosis.*
- *Clinicians may have concerns about their ability to manage PD patients in crisis.*

- *Clinicians may have undue concern about liability in the management of PD patients' crises.*
- *Polypharmacy or aimless unstructured psychotherapies may reflect clinicians' unexplored countertransference to certain PD patients.*

Why should borderline personality disorder be "the diagnosis doctors fear most" as described by the lay press? [14] Why do even conscientious clinicians seem prone to avoid making a personality disorder diagnosis? Why do clinicians who strongly support the modern trend away from patriarchal, authoritarian medical practices routinely withhold from patients a reliably made personality disorder diagnoses [15]?

The answers to these questions are complex and multiply determined. The clinician's response to PD patients' crises may be one essential element of this oft-cited chronic and negative countertransference pattern. To be sure, PD pathology can add an element of urgency and uncertainty to any situation. Clinicians may recoil from this possibility and "vow" to avoid treatment of PD patients, although this may be unrealistic for many providers. Alternatively, clinicians may unconsciously avoid identifying PD symptoms. For example, the psychiatrist who identifies recurrent affective dysregulation and threats of suicide as a "rapid cycling" mood disturbance, or the psychologist who accepts a narcissistic patient's chronic underperformance at work as evidence of an Attention Deficit Disorder even if symptoms inventories do not support such a diagnosis.

Many clinicians may feel too inexperienced to identify and treat personality disorders. The closure of many hospitals' long-term treatment units has reduced opportunities for trainees and recent graduates to work with patients with severe personality disorders in safe, well-supervised settings. Some clinicians feel their training may have given them limited exposure to the current evidence-based treatments available or exposure to only one element of a treatment, for example, a dialectical behavior therapy (DBT) skills group focused on mindfulness, but without the other three elements of telephone coaching, individual treatment, and peer supervision.

Treating patients with PDs does require additional focus on risk management issues, but these risks are not reduced by ignoring the symptoms or calling them something else. Clinicians may fear they are increasing their risk of liability if they identify PD symptoms and engage their patients in a discussion of the PD diagnosis. There is no data to support this concern, but it persists in many clinical settings [16]. Ignorance about PDs and failure to investigate PD symptoms and engage patients and families in proactive psychoeducation may, in fact, be a more likely path to increased liability exposure.

Clinicians' aversion to PD patients and their efforts to either minimize or ignore PD symptoms may be, in part, responsible for two widely described and reviled phenomena of contemporary practice: extended, aimless psychotherapies and complicated, ineffective polypharmacy. The TFP attitude would question a superficially supportive psychotherapy of a patient unable to move forward in the major spheres of adult life of meaningful work and intimate relations. In TFP such a treatment would be suspect for a chronic countertransference enactment of a therapist fearful of the patient's aggression covertly conveying acceptance of the patient's passivity and resignation. In a similar vein, ineffective, complex polypharmacy with prominent side effects (weight gain, hypersomnia) in a borderline patient could be interpreted as a reflection of the patient's desire to be cared for by a benevolent prescriber without having to make an effort or the clinician's unexplored aggression in response to a frustrating patient.

Mrs. M.'s Psychiatrist is Reluctant to Make a Diagnosis of Borderline Personality Disorder, Fearing It Would "Open a Can of Worms"

Clinical vignette: Mrs. M. is a 30-year-old married woman, working as a school principal, who has been under the care of a psychiatrist she sees monthly for 30-minute

(continued)

(continued)

"medication checks" for the past 4 years. She has been given a variety of diagnoses by this psychiatrist including attention deficit disorder, cyclothymia, and generalized anxiety disorder. She has significant mood instability almost always in the context of interpersonal conflict with her sister or her parents, intermittent threats of suicide, and periods of impulsivity including the initiation of an affair with her tennis coach. Mrs. M.'s psychiatrist has made multiple medication changes over time, resulting in a complicated medication regimen including two antidepressants, a stimulant, a mood stabilizer, an atypical antipsychotic medication, and a sedative-hypnotic medication for chronic sleep disturbance.

Mrs. M. becomes markedly suicidal after a rejection by her tennis coach and tells her parents she plans to follow through with her threats of suicide by walking into traffic. This precipitates an emergency family meeting with her psychiatrist and family, and referral to Ms. D., a TFP-trained social worker, for a more frequent psychotherapy to complement her ongoing monthly psychiatric visits.

Ms. D. completes a three-session evaluation and feels confident in conveying to Mrs. M. and to Mrs. M.'s psychiatrist her diagnostic impression that includes a primary borderline personality disorder diagnosis. Ms. D. outlines for Mrs. M. a plan to review with her psychiatrist her diagnostic impression and her suggestion of simplifying her medication regimen over time and focusing on individual psychotherapy and family psychoeducation about BPD. Mrs. M.'s psychiatrist acknowledges to Ms. D. that he had considered exploring a personality disorder diagnosis at different points but feared the format they had in place of brief monthly meetings would not allow such exploration. He describes feeling "barely able to manage making medication changes with each new crisis" and concerned that discussion of PD symptoms

(continued)

(continued)

"would have opened a can of worms." Ms. D. notes that after describing BPD to Mrs. M. and suggesting this single diagnosis might be more accurate that the multiple diagnoses she had received, Mrs. M. did not explode but appeared open to hearing about the diagnosis, reflecting, "I'd heard about borderline and sometimes wondered if I might have it," and asked Ms. D. a series of thoughtful questions about the disorder's treatments and prognosis.

Take Home Point: Exploration of borderline personality disorder symptoms and frank discussion with a patient about a reliably made diagnosis can be to the patient's advantage.

3.5   TFP Principles in Managing PD Patients in Crisis

- *TFP accepts that speculation about personality disorder diagnoses may be required at times with incomplete information.*
- *TFP allows the clinician to think beyond arbitrary descriptive psychiatry cutoffs in assessing personality disorder pathology.*
- *TFP alerts the clinician to consider a patient's use of splitting-based defenses and how those defenses are expressed in the patient's life and any treatment setting.*
- *TFP interventions often begin with accepting confusion and attempting to contain the patient by "naming the actors."*
- *The patient in crisis will prompt the TFP-trained clinician to consider the dominant object relations dyad in evidence and to observe for its likely reversal.*

TFP's use of the structural interview as a foundation for its approach dictates that clinicians consider personality organization and possible personality disorder symptoms from the outset. This approach may differ from a long held belief that personality disorders cannot be reliably diagnosed until all other major psychiatric conditions are in remission. That attitude was derived from a number of historical factors: a belief that personality disorder diagnoses are *uniquely* lacking in validity, an expectation that personality disorder pathology is fixed and unresponsive to treatment, and the idea that personality disorder diagnoses may reflect clinicians' unexplored antipathy to particular patients [17, 18].

The TFP approach accepts that the clinician may need to consider personality organization and personality disorder traits with incomplete information. TFP also encourages clinicians to think beyond the current DSM-5 categories with its arbitrary cutoffs of symptom counts. TFP's approach is consistent with the emerging hybrid categorical-dimensional approach to personality disorder diagnosis in the DSM-5 appendix (Sect. 3.4) [19]. Research on the clinical significance of even *one* BPD symptom further supports the TFP approach to diagnostic assessment [20].

The TFP assessment process orients the clinician to the patient's level of psychological organization. This is informed by the clinician's assessment of the patient's predominant defensive operations, which in turn alerts the clinician to the possibility of clinical crises going forward. Appreciation of the dominance of splitting-based defenses alerts the clinician to the high likelihood of crises of various kinds emerging in the evaluation process and the psychotherapy. Understanding the use of splitting-based defenses orients the clinician to expect certain, specific object relations dyads (and their inverses) likely to emerge in treatment, reflected in what the patient says, how the patient behaves, and how the clinician feels.

The BPO patient's use of splitting-based defenses may precipitate crises in the following ways:

Idealization/Devaluation: Primitive idealization and devaluation reflect the patient's experience of others as either

entirely good or entirely bad. The patient may initially experience the therapist as entirely good, as a powerful protector
against another person experienced as entirely bad (e.g., an
estranged spouse). An appreciation of this defensive pattern
would alert the clinician to the high risk for an eventual rapid
and stark reversal in this experience of others. The clinician
could anticipate a crisis, possibly a threat to end treatment,
when the patient's primitive idealization shifts abruptly to an
experience of the therapist as totally bad as soon as a disap-
pointment with him or her arises.

Projection/Projective Identification: In projection, the patient
ascribes some aspect of his or her internal state to an external
source. For example, a harshly self-critical patient may
ascribe aspects of this self-criticism to another individual and
react accordingly. This phenomenon can be seen in the assessment of a patient who is "certain" that some specific group
harbors negative, even denigrating, feelings toward her. In
the transference this may emerge as a patient's certainty that
the therapist has disdain for some aspect of the patient
(appearance, background, education) the patient herself feels
poorly about. It is easy to imagine how this process of pro-
jecting these negative feelings onto others could precipitate
crises. One scenario is that the BPD patient unhappy with her
physical appearance gets an entry-level job and quits abruptly
after the first week "because everybody in the office was
looking down at me because I'm overweight."

Denial: The patient managing conflict by keeping out of
awareness emotions related to serious, important concerns
may be using denial as a defense. The patient who does not
have an appropriate emotional reaction to certain external
realities may be at risk when it is no longer possible to keep
these realities at bay. For example, the patient who cannot
accept the realities of his or her finances may face a crisis in
treatment at the end of the month when presented with the
bill. The power of denial can lead patients to agree without
hesitation to a certain fee for treatment, only to realize
quickly that the responsibility for the fee isn't feasible.

Omnipotent Control: The defense of omnipotent control allows the patient to feel, and sometimes be, in control of others who are experienced as either positive (in an idealized way) or negative (and therefore a potential source of persecution or retaliation). The patient keeping the object/other in a "positive" light perpetuates a wish for an ideal, benevolent figure. The patient keeping the object/other in a "negative" light can protect the patient from the risk of his or her own aggressive affect. It is easy to imagine how a crisis could arise when the patient's controlling style of relating is challenged. The collision between the patient's expression of omnipotent control and the clinician's requirement for self-protection is often the point of crisis which leads the clinician to begin to consider a severe PD diagnosis. For example, the therapist who assumes care for a borderline patient who has "failed" multiple prior treatments finds herself acting in an unusually accommodating way with scheduling. The therapist does not hold to her cancellation policy with this patient and often allows sessions to go on a half hour or even an hour longer than had been scheduled. In this scenario the patient's expression of omnipotent control, out of awareness of both parties, perpetuates the patient's experience of the therapist as entirely positive, at least for awhile. Inevitably a crisis arises and then the therapist can no longer accommodate the patient in a way that maintains a purely positive transference. When the therapist has a work commitment requiring she end the session on time (self-protection), the patient becomes hurt and angry as the patient's omnipotent control of the therapist is challenged (loss of idealized, benevolent figure).

The clinician encountering the patient in crisis will often feel compelled to actively organize the material shared by the patient into a clear formulation in an effort to de-escalate the situation. This effort is understandable but may bypass empathizing with the complexity of the patient's internal experience. The TFP-trained clinician encountering a BPO or BPD patient in crisis will accept the expectable confusion conveyed by the patient and aim not to organize the patient's complaints or respond to those complaints with immediate solutions but will rather aim to contain the situation by "naming the actors" or translating the content conveyed into a rough estimation of the dominant object relations at play.

"Naming the actors" in a crisis situation involves describing the object relations dyad most available to the patient at that time. Often this dyad reflects the patient's experience as vulnerable or powerless, feeling aggrieved or angry at the hands of a punitive or harmful victimizer. While there are variations on these themes, the process of "naming the actors" allows the therapist to convey some sense of understanding about how the patient is feeling, which often has a powerful containing effect.

The next step after "naming the actors" is to observe for oscillation, or reversal of roles, within the dominant object relations dyad, when "the shoe is on the other foot" and the patient who presents as powerless or vulnerable is observed as treating others in ways similar to those described in the complaint of mistreatment. This intervention serves to bring into the patient's awareness, however briefly, a critical aspect of behavior (in this case a pattern of aggressive mistreatment toward another) the patient does not "own."

Dr. S. Uses Her Countertransference to Help Guide Treatment of a "Difficult Patient" in the Emergency Department

Clinical vignette: Dr. S. is an attending psychiatrist in a busy big city psychiatric emergency room. The emergency room triage department is staffed by social workers who screen the patients on their arrival. Dr. S. is in the process of assessing a number of different patients when she is paged by the triage unit social worker to come at once to meet with Ms. L., who is threatening to contact hospital administration if she is not seen immediately. Dr. S. knew only that Ms. L. was a local attorney who had taken an overdose of sleeping medication she was describing as "a mistake" and wanted to leave that hospi-

(continued)

(continued)

tal as soon as possible. The social worker added that records indicated Ms. L. had had a similar episode the previous year and with coordination with her psychiatrist was discharged from the emergency department after an overnight stay.

Dr. S. considered herself a full-time psychiatric emergency clinician but had made a point of taking a 1-day course in TFP at the annual psychiatry meetings because of her concerns about her ability to manage patients with personality disorder symptoms in the emergency room setting. She did not know, in fact, if Ms. L. carried a personality disorder diagnosis but sensed from the social worker's account of the prior emergency department visit that this might be possible.

Dr. S. was already aware of her countertransference (irritation, dread) at having to see Ms. L. emergently. She also noted the social worker's uncharacteristic anxiety as she conveyed the urgency of having Ms. L. seen out of turn. Dr. S. found Ms. L. pacing in her room looking impatient and angry. When Dr. S. introduced herself, Ms. L. interrupted her stating: "You need to get me out of here now! This is a mistake and I'll make a lot of trouble for you if I miss work tomorrow!"

Dr. S. was aware of her motivation to respond defensively, answering "You're the one who started this by taking the overdose!," but she resisted doing so and contemplated what she imagined was the dominant object relations dyad (powerful doctor, vulnerable patient) and the likely inverse in play (demanding patient, fearful clinicians). Dr. S. hoped that by containing Mr. L.'s affect, she could then fulfill her professional responsibility to collect enough material to make a decision about whether it was, in fact, safe to let Ms. L. go home.

(continued)

(continued)

Dr. S. began by naming the actors: "It seems you're worried I'm indifferent to your concerns and that you'll suffer because of my indifference." Ms. L. shook her head in agreement: "You're damned right! I've been waiting here most of the night and if I wait all night I'll miss an important appointment in the morning!" Dr. S. responded: "You've been focused on how I'm so powerful here and you're so vulnerable, but I'm aware that you're the one raising her voice and speaking in a threatening way. I'd like to get a full history so that we can determine what's happened and how to help you stay safe." Ms. L. became less aggressive and more cooperative in response to this exchange with Dr. S.; they were able to complete the evaluation in a timely manner, and Dr. S. was able to discharge Ms. L. home with confidence.

Take Home Point: Using the intervention of "naming the actors" can convey to patients an experience of being understood and help clinicians de-escalate crisis situations.

3.6   PD Crisis Management in Mental Health and Medical Systems

- *PD patients will often first present to clinicians in crisis.*
- *Clinicians may not be aware of PD symptoms until patients are in crisis.*
- *PD patients in crisis will be found throughout mental health and medical settings.*
- *PD patients in crisis may require assessment for changes in level of care or type of care.*

Many clinicians will feel comfortable identifying PD symptoms only in the most severely disturbed patients. These clinicians may be familiar with a small group of patients known for recurrent suicidality, emergency room visits, or inpatient hospitalizations. These clinicians therefore will be less likely to appreciate PD in other settings such as routine outpatient psychiatric care or outpatient or inpatient medical services.

Very often clinicians will not begin to think about PD symptoms until a patient in a routine setting is in crisis. These crises may come as a surprise to the clinician and may require extra attention and efforts from the staff of an outpatient clinic or office setting or inpatient staff including nurses and administrators. The PD patient may present with a "self-defined" crisis. In the outpatient psychiatric setting, this might be an urgent need for medication refills, an abrupt onset of suicidal or homicidal feelings, or the desire to switch treaters emergently. In medical settings the PD patient may present in crisis related to escalating somatic symptoms, complaints about staff, or noncompliance including threats to leave the hospital "against medical advice." (See Chap. 7 for a full discussion of treating PD patients in Primary Care Medicine settings.)

Some crises will require prompt referral to specialized crisis care settings such as the emergency room. In these cases a clinician will act immediately to insure conditions of safety and only then pause to fully reflect on the specific meaning of the crisis in terms of diagnostic understanding, insight into the patient's dynamics, and treatment planning. In many other cases the clinician is compelled to weigh the risks and benefits of recommending to patients a change in the level of care provided. These recommendations can require complex calculations, assessing the safety of the patient and the therapist, understanding the meanings for the patient in changing the level of care, and considering the potential pitfalls associated with such changes.

The continuum of psychiatric services ranges from typical outpatient individual office or clinic-based treatments to intermediate higher levels of care such as partial hospital or intensive outpatient programs to residential treatment programs and hospital-based settings including emergency departments and inpatient psychiatric units. The TFP therapist treating the PD patient in crisis is always asking: What do I need to do to make sure the patient is safe? What do I need to do to insure I feel safe? How does this current "crisis" reflect the patient's dominant object relations? What are the steps required to then get the treatment "back on track" after this disruption?

The extensive literature on hospitalization for patients with BPD concludes that there are certain situations necessitating inpatient treatment and other scenarios associated with considerable risks in doing so [21]. Experts have endorsed hospitalization for the following: new onset frank psychosis, worsening of a co-occurring mood disorder not manageable as an outpatient, or reconsideration of the overall treatment plan for a patient following a near-lethal suicide attempt. On the other hand, experts have concluded that clinicians may sometimes opt for hospitalization in situations where their countertransferential anxiety overrides their understanding of the likely risks and benefits of hospitalization.

The potential risks associated with hospitalization of PD patients have been well described. The wish for hospitalization can sometimes reflect the patient's desire to shed responsibilities and to be cared for by an infinitely attentive staff. The reality of today's inpatient psychiatric unit will often come as a rude shock to patients who will abruptly shift from wanting immediate admission to wanting immediate discharge. Hospitalizations can disrupt a patient's studies or employment, often causing problems lasting many months following even a brief inpatient stay. Individual psychotherapy is disrupted as well. TFP stresses the therapist's limited involvement with a patient in the emergency room or inpatient unit; the TFP therapist will not offer daily "sessions" to the hospitalized patient but will reiterate the advance directive of the TFP contract that the patient will be expected to follow the recommendations of the emergency room and inpatient clinicians without interference by the primary therapist. Patients sometimes criticize the TFP therapist for "getting out of the picture when the going gets tough." To counter this impression (a transference), the therapist makes clear during the contracting phase that the role of exploratory therapist is not compatible with that of crisis manager and that it detracts from therapy to blur these roles. The therapist who becomes involved in crisis management often unwittingly rewards the crisis behavior with extra attention – a pattern which should be avoided.

Partial hospital or intensive outpatient programs are sometimes a reasonable recommendation for PD patients with escalating symptoms. In TFP such a recommendation might be appropriate when the patient has the onset of symptoms that cannot be effectively managed by one clinician or a split treatment, requiring a program, often for an interim period, before the patient returns to TFP. For the patient with a substance use disorder whose relapse cannot be managed without comprehensive care, a referral to a higher level of care can insure the patient accesses appropriate treatment toward consolidated sobriety before returning to TFP. Similarly, the eating disorder patient whose symptoms escalate may require a program with on-site CBT, nutritional counseling, and medicine liaison. Again, the patient would be reevaluated for TFP when the level of eating disorder symptomatology no longer threatens the patient's ability to engage effectively in psychotherapy. After the behavioral symptomatology is under adequate control, the TFP therapist can get back to helping the patient achieve the identity integration that is central to achieving the goals of satisfaction in the areas of work/vocation and relationships/love.

Dr. J. Identifies Treatment-Interfering Substance Use Requiring a Temporary Change in the TFP Treatment Frame

Clinical vignette: Dr. J., a psychologist, has begun TFP treatment with a new patient, Laura, a 25-year-old dancer who had been in treatment for eating, mood, and alcohol

(continued)

(continued)

use disorder symptoms during much of her adolescence. Dr. J. feels comfortable discussing the diagnosis of BPD she has made with Laura at the outset of their treatment, and Laura agrees that the BPD symptoms described accurately reflect her experience.

Dr. J. accepts Laura's account of her current alcohol use, by her reports a significant reduction following years in college of weekly binge drinking to blackout and multiple arrests for driving while intoxicated. After the third month of treatment, Laura begins to cancel frequently, complaining of poor sleep and difficulty "getting out of the house." After Laura's third canceled appointment, Dr. J. asks Laura directly about her alcohol use. Laura reports that the stress of work has led her to drink frequently to the point of intoxication. At their next meeting, Dr. J. smells alcohol on Laura's breath, and Laura discloses that she has begun drinking daily in the morning to manage her anxiety.

Dr. J. concludes that Laura's alcohol use pattern has made effective individual psychotherapy impossible at this time. She outlines for Laura a plan for suspension of their TFP treatment, and she refers Laura to a program first for alcohol detoxification and then for specialized outpatient alcohol use disorder treatment.

After 6 months of sobriety, Laura contacts Dr. J. to restart their TFP treatment. Laura and Dr. J. review her ongoing adjunctive treatment (12-step group participation and periodic meetings with an addiction psychiatrist). They restart treatment with a plan for active communication between Dr. J. and Laura's addiction psychiatrist.

Take Home Point: The therapist will need to assess for treatment-threatening behaviors and may feel compelled to temporarily suspend TFP if necessary.

3.7   TFP Principles Can Aid Risk Management Efforts

> - *TFP principles reinforce clinicians' monitoring of exceptions made to standard practice.*
> - *TFP principles can help clinicians avoid unnecessary crisis-generated pharmacotherapy (polypharmacy, unusual dosing or supplies).*
> - *TFP principles reinforce vigilance about boundary violations with PD patients.*
> - *TFP principles reinforce attention to countertransference-induced distancing from PD patients.*

TFP training is a useful and practical addition to general risk management practices. Because TFP was developed for PD patients, its approach integrates attitudes and practices preparing clinicians for some of the most challenging risk management predicaments.

The TFP emphasis on exploration of countertransference adds to the standard risk management attitude about self-monitoring for unusual or extraordinary measures in patient care. Attentions to countertransference enactments involving boundary violations, patient abandonment, or dangerous prescribing practices are some of the well-described medico-legal pitfalls in treatment of BPD [22]. TFP's strong endorsement of the use of consultation for clinicians feeling overwhelmed or unduly anxious is another useful risk management intervention.

The TFP attitude posits that there is meaning for the patient in receiving prescriptions. This attitude prompts prescribers to move beyond a "medical model" approach – the patient has these symptoms, I will prescribe a medication to address it – to one actively speculating about the activated dyad at a particular time. A prescriber may feel pressured to use higher than recommended doses of a medication or to prescribe larger supplies or more refills in response to the patient pulling for "special treatment" from an idealized caregiver and creating the feeling that anything less than special treatment confirms that the therapist is negligent. TFP principles will compel the prescriber to ask: Why am I making an exception to my usual practice in this case? What is the underlying dyad? What are my countertransferential reactions?

Similarly, the therapist who finds himself or herself making "heroic" interventions to advocate for a patient or changing practice habits to accommodate a patient will consider the dyads likely contributing to such exceptions. The therapist may reflect: Am I making these exceptions because I can't tolerate the patient shifting from an idealized experience of me to one marked by devaluation with associated anger? The TFP attitude of expecting and accepting negativity in the transference can prevent boundary violations emerging from the clinician's unconscious motivation to stay idealized. Much clinical experience has shown that even highly skilled therapists often engage in acting out (e.g., making exceptions) in their treatment of PD patients to avoid accusations from patients that the clinician is a "bad" therapist or person, a sentiment often expressed as part of a negative transference.

The TFP contract implicitly addresses the risk for patient abandonment. While borderline patients' highly variable dropout rate from treatment has been documented for years, it is also true that many therapists, directly or indirectly, find ways of ending therapy with a PD patient [23]. Novice clinicians often find themselves at risk for abruptly severing ties with a patient they have come to experience as intrusive, destructive, or uncooperative. The TFP contract explores those contingencies *in advance* and sets up parameters to work with them. The risks associated with the therapist's impulsive termination of a patient, often in an affectively charged moment in the treatment, are therefore limited.

Dr. Y. Becomes Concerned about the Risk of Her Colleague's Countertransference-Induced Boundary Violations

Clinical vignette: Dr. Y. is a psychiatrist at a university counseling center. She often supervises other clinicians providing psychotherapy to students as part of her responsibilities. During her residency Dr. Y. learned about TFP from a supervisor and treated one case in her fourth year of training using an "applied TFP" approach.

Ms. S. is a social worker new to the counseling center who presents a case to Dr. Y. of Melanie, a college freshman who came for treatment with symptoms of dysphoria, loneliness, and passive suicidality. Ms. S. is impassioned in her advocacy for this student, feeling strongly that one professor had mistreated the student by giving her a low grade and sharing Melanie's anger at her parents after they forbid her from using marijuana, which she said she needed to relax while home on vacation. Ms. S. implores Dr. Y. to see Melanie in her "crisis" slot, believing she should be started on antidepressant medication immediately.

Dr. Y. meets with Melanie but defers starting medication until she can obtain baseline laboratory testing. The following day Ms. S. leaves the staff meeting to take an emergency call from Melanie and then schedules a meeting with Melanie at the end of the day after the clinic is officially closed. Later that evening Ms. S. texts Dr. Y. to let her know that she is on her way to Melanie's dorm room after the student had called her "hysterical and threatening."

Dr. Y. invokes her TFP training in speculating about the countertransference reaction she has identified in Ms. S. She is able to contact Ms. S. and to share with her certain basic risk management points as well as TFP-informed speculation about the dominant dyad at play

(continued)

(continued)

(suffering patient and idealized nurturing and available parental figure) and the potential for shifts in this dyad. Dr. Y. is able to convince Ms. S. to follow clinic protocol, involving Melanie's resident advisor first, then the Dean's Office, before meeting next with Melanie during regular office hours at the clinic with Dr. Y., as well as the clinic director, present.

Take Home Point: Active monitoring of countertransference as part of the TFP approach to treating patients with personality disorder pathology in crisis is a good risk management tool.

References

1. Sansone RA, Sansone LA. Responses of mental health clinicians to patients with borderline personality disorder. Innov Clin Neurosci. 2013;10(5–6):39–43.
2. Lewis G, Appleby L. Personality disorder: the patients psychiatrists dislike. Br J Psychiatr. 1988;153(1):44–9.
3. American Psychiatric Association. Diagnostic and statistical manual of mental disorders. 5th ed. Washington, DC: American Psychiatric Press; 2013.
4. Zerbo E, Cohen S, Bielska W, Caligor E. Transference-focused psychotherapy in the general psychiatry residency: a useful and applicable model for residents in acute clinical settings. Psychodyn Psychiatry. 2013;41(1):163–81.
5. Ricke AK, Lee MJ, Chambers JE. The difficult patient: borderline personality disorder in the obstetrical and gynecological patient. Obstet Gynecol Surv. 2012;67(8):495–502.
6. Dubovsky AN, Kiefer MM. Borderline personality disorder in the primary care settings. Med Clin. 2014;98(5):1049–64.
7. Sansone R, Kay J, Anderson J. Resident didactic education in borderline personality disorder: is it sufficient? Acad Psychiatr. 2013;37(4):287–8.
8. Paris J. Why psychiatrists are reluctant to diagnose borderline personality disorder. Psychiatry. 2007;4(1):35–9.

9. Zimmerman M, Mattia JI. Differences between clinical and research practices in diagnosis borderline personality disorder. Am J Psychiatr. 1999;156:1570–4.
10. Paris J. Is hospitalization useful for suicidal patients with borderline personality disorder? J Pers Disord. 2004;18:240–7.
11. Applebaum PS, Gutheil TF. Clinical handbook of psychiatry and the law. 4th ed. Philadelphia: Lippincott Williams & Wilkins; 2007.
12. Yeomans FE, Selzer MA, Clarkin JF. Treating the borderline patient: a contract-based approach. New York: Basic Books; 1992.
13. Gunderson JG, Ridolfi ME. Borderline personality disorder: suicide and self-mutilation. Ann NY Acad Sci. 2001;932:61–73.
14. Cloud J. Borderline personality: the disorder doctors fear the most. Time Mag. 2009;173(2):42–6.
15. Lequesne ER, Hersh RG. Disclosure of a borderline personality diagnosis. J Psychiatr Pract. 2004;10:170–6.
16. Zanarini MC, Frankenburg FR. A preliminary, randomized trial of psychoeducation for women with borderline personality disorder. J Pers Disord. 2008;22(3):284–90.
17. Vaillant GE. The beginning of wisdom is never calling a patient a borderline; or the clinical management of immature defenses in the treatment of individuals with personality disorders. J Psychother Pract Res. 1992;1(2):117–34.
18. Akiskal HS, Chen SE, Davis GC, Puzantian VR, Kashgarian M, Bolinger JM. Borderline: an adjunctive in search of a noun. J Clin Psychiatr. 1985;46(2):41–8.
19. Skodol AE, Morey LC, Bender DS, Oldham JM. The alternative DSM-5 model for personality disorders: a clinical application. Am J Psychiatr. 2015;172(7):606–13.
20. Zimmerman M, Chelminski I, Young D, Dalrymple K, Martinez J. Does the presence of one feature of borderline personality disorder have clinical significance? Implications for dimensional ratings of personality disorders. J Clin Psychiatr. 2012;73(1):8–12.
21. Paris J. Treatment of borderline personality disorder: a guide to evidence-based practice. New York: Guilford Press; 2008.
22. Gutheil TG. Medicolegal pitfalls in the treatment of borderline patients. Am J Psychiatr. 1985;142:9–14.
23. Barnicot K, Katsakou C, Marougka S, Priebe S. Treatment completion in psychotherapy for borderline personality disorder: a systemic review and meta-analysis. Acta Psychiatr Scand. 2011;123(5):327–8.

Chapter 4
Transference-Focused Psychotherapy (TFP) Principles in Work with the Families of Patients with Severe Personality Disorders

1. *TFP principles often lead to more clinician contact with families (parents or spouse/partner) than would be expected in a traditional psychoanalytic psychotherapy.*
2. *TFP clinicians will suggest a family meeting in many cases as part of the assessment process and will almost always require one (and follow-up meetings if indicated) if family members are caring for the patient in practical ways (e.g., paying for the treatment or parents providing housing for the adult patient).*
3. *TFP openness about PD diagnoses and prognosis extends to dialogue with families.*
4. *Family involvement requires explicit discussion about TFP and ways it differs from other treatments including TFP's limits on certain treatment-interfering behaviors.*
5. *TFP supports families in helping them deal with patients' ways of controlling through threats of self-harm, non-compliance, and passivity.*

(continued)

© Springer International Publishing Switzerland 2016 91
R.G. Hersh et al., *Fundamentals of Transference-Focused Psychotherapy*, DOI 10.1007/978-3-319-44091-0_4

(continued)

6. *Family psychoeducation about the goal of medication reduction, particularly if recruited by patients to see this as "depriving."*
7. *TFP principles informing family involvement are useful risk management tools.*

4.1   Introduction

While TFP was developed as an individual psychodynamic psychotherapy with its roots in classical psychoanalytic theory, its approach to family engagement differs significantly from the tradition of the inviolate patient-therapist dyad [1]. TFP's appreciation of defensive operations commonly utilized by patients operating on a borderline level dictates a more engaged, open attitude with family members, including parents, spouses, and children. Since the acting out of intense affects and psychological conflicts is not limited to discreet actions but can occur in the way the patient leads his/her life, it is logical to engage the people who are involved in the patient's day-to-day life in a discussion of how the patient's way of relating to them, and vice versa, might need to be addressed as part of the therapeutic process. In TFP, family involvement is not seen as a "last resort" intervention for patients in crisis, but rather an integrated set of interventions in the treatment, consistent with other contemporary theoretical approaches to personality disorder treatment stressing the potential benefits of family involvement [2].

In TFP a meeting with family members as part of the assessment process is considered highly desirable in most cases and almost always mandatory when the family members are involved in practical ways, such as paying for the patient's treatment. The goals of this meeting are many:

obtaining parallel information, demystifying the therapy and the therapist; preemptively addressing the possiblity of an emerging "split" between the family and the therapist; challenging pathological patterns of dependence; and reinforcing the "reality" of the patient's reliance on family financial support when indicated. The initial meeting may need to be followed by periodic family meetings in certain cases, particularly with patients with prominent dishonesty and antisocial traits.

As with all of the other evidence-based treatments for BPD, TFP endorses the explicit discussion with patients and families about the personality disorder diagnosis and its prognosis [3–6]. Because TFP has built into its patient contract the requirement for paid work, volunteer work, or meaningful school involvement, the TFP therapist is often obligated to explain to families the distinction between disabling conditions (e.g., treatment-resistant depression, chronic and debilitating medical conditions) and resistance to meaningful activity resulting from character pathology. The therapist may also explain the therapeutic value of a structured activity involving others, both in terms of what it brings up for discussion in therapy and ultimately the sense of satisfaction it can provide. TFP's appreciation of common object relations dyads identified in BPO patients anticipates that some families will be influenced by patients to experience the therapist as callous or unrealistic in expecting work or school as part of their treatment.

The TFP contracting phase includes active exploration of potentially treatment-interfering behaviors. In fact, TFP can require a substance-using patient to have a protracted period of sobriety or an eating disorder patient to have a weight minimum determined by an internist before beginning psychotherapy. These stipulations may be experienced by families as unfair or arbitrary. Again, these specifics of the TFP model can make family involvement essential if not obligatory.

Many families find themselves struggling with patients' use of defensive omnipotent control, while very few of these families are familiar with this concept. In these situations, patients manage, through their actions, to exert control over family members, leaving them frustrated, frightened, or resigned. All therapy models for families with BPD patients stress confrontation of this pattern; TFP adds a more specific and direct approach to some patients' passive exploitation and "secondary gain."

For families accustomed to treaters with "on call" availability, the TFP model of limited intersession contact may come as a surprise. Families may join patients who hear this aspect of the TFP contract, along with discussion in advance of the therapist's purposeful *absence* in the decision-making process in emergency rooms and inpatient units, as uncaring or delinquent. The TFP therapist involves families early in the treatment to prepare them for what might happen. This is particularly important with chronically suicidal patients who may use their suicidality in a way that is provocative and aggressive or seeks to increase contact. The therapist helps the family understand the distinction between in-depth exploratory therapy, which has the goal of effecting changes in the personality and satisfaction in work and love, and emergency services, which deal with crises but do not provide the opportunity for working toward deep change.

Families may understandably be concerned and confused about patient suicidality. Families may have difficulty distinguishing between chronic and acute suicidality, compelling treaters to help them distinguish between the two. Some PD patients will threaten suicide and non-suicidal self-injurious behavior reflecting ego-syntonic aggression – as part of a way of expressing angry and hostile feelings – further complicating the clinician's task of assessing suicidality and managing its effects on family members.

Accruing evidence supports an increasingly focused and limited role for psychotropic medications in the treatment of most personality disorders [7]. This perspective may be disconcerting to families, particularly in cases when prior clinicians have stressed the contribution of co-occurring conditions or conveyed unrealistic hopes for the effectiveness of medications. Patients who experience polypharmacy as gratifying will resist simplification of their medication regimen even if the regimen is not particularly effective. Families may be recruited by patients to protest medication reductions, which requires prescribers to explain in detail their diagnostic thinking, risks and benefits of medication trials, and the likely psychodynamics underlying this polypharmacy.

TFP requires patients to engage in some kind of meaningful work or school experience as a prerequisite for psychotherapy. This requirement correlates closely with the structural interview's attention to a range of behaviors from subtle, passive exploitation to frank sociopathy. The structural interview stresses details such as the patient's work history, finances, and sources of financial support, which can be easily overlooked in a standard "medical model" assessment. We remind the reader, and the family, again that the patient's way of leading his or her life can be part of a pathological dynamic. Certain patients with borderline, narcissistic, dependent, or hypochondriacal personality traits will derive "secondary gain" from their conditions, often leading to passive lifestyles and continued family support into adulthood. Families can become inured to this phenomenon and react with alarm when the clinician proposes setting a limit of some kind on this support. Yet, in some cases, there is virtually no hope for change without such a limit. TFP principles will guide the clinician to help families reflect on and address the difference between what a patient "can't" and "won't" do in this context. Clinicians are often dependent on families to take action by supporting limit setting and may be thwarted by families unable to do so.

Many clinicians fear working with patients with moderate to severe personality disorder symptoms will put them at risk for increased liability. While the liability incurred in treating PD patient may be higher than for most psychiatric patients, the literature suggests the risk is low or perhaps negligible for experienced clinicians [8]. Liability risks are closely associated with unexamined aspects of the clinicians' countertransference which can lead to boundary violations, abandonment, or "heroic" interventions. TFP training's openness to family involvement can mitigate the risks described by "opening up" the patient-therapist dyad. The family's familiarity with the clinician and explicit family psychoeducation, including discussion of morbidity and mortality risks, are other useful risk management interventions.

4.2   TFP Attitudes Toward Family Involvement

- *TFP will generally support more family contact than in a traditional psychoanalytic psychotherapy.*
- *Clinician contact with family implicitly confronts some patients' assumptions that individual psychotherapy, by definition, remains a "closed system."*
- *Clinician contact with family may stimulate paranoia in the transference that the TFP therapist will need to explore.*
- *TFP clinicians will be open to ongoing family support or treatment with other treaters.*

Although TFP is a psychotherapy derived from psychoanalytic theory, its attitude toward family involvement differs significantly from traditional psychoanalysis or psychoanalytic psychotherapy. TFP's attitude about family involvement results directly from an understanding of the predominant defenses associated with BPO or BPD. With regard to family involvement, TFP is closely aligned with the other evidence-based treatments for BPD and with the developing and influential advocacy organization movement supported by families of individuals with BPD [9, 10].

Some patients may come to TFP from psychotherapies not open to family involvement, hewing to a more traditional pattern of "protecting" the patient-therapist dyad from outside influences. While this model may be of use to many patients, exclusion of family involvement for many patients with BPO or BPD may reflect a countertransferential collusion with the patient's expression of omnipotent control. A typical example of this could be the following: An adult patient has convinced her family that she is too ill to work and requires family monetary support while in an open-ended individual psychotherapy. The therapist in this case has not been open to family involvement, accepting the patient's account of hostile, intrusive parents who nonetheless support the adult patient financially. A new TFP-trained therapist assumes some kind of family involvement in the treatment, given the family's active financial involvement. The new therapist presents this to the patient in the assessment and contracting phase causing the patient consternation understood by the therapist as emerging paranoia in the transference.

How could the subject of family involvement trigger a paranoid reaction in the transference? As described, family involvement implicitly confronts frequently observed dominant dyads in BPO and BPD including sadistic parents and vulnerable patient alternating with controlling patient and powerless parents. Since the object relations dyads in the patient's mind – made up of representations of self and other in specific relationship patterns – can determine the patient's experience of the world around her, she may genuinely see her parents as sadistic and controlling and could think the therapist was an agent of their control. The challenge for the therapist is to establish enough of an alliance with the patient to explore this view as the patient is experiencing it. Family involvement may also feel threatening to the more sociopathic patient who has developed a parasitic relationship with family. In that case the patient may rightly be concerned that a TFP approach will directly confront this parasitism in a way not done in the patient's prior supportive psychotherapy.

There are, of course, some cases where family involvement may not be appropriate. Clinicians may be required to do extensive investigation with patients with trauma histories before feeling comfortable enough to recommend family contact. These situations require careful deliberation on a case-by-case basis, weighing the potential benefits of family involvement with the risks of exacerbating a trauma-associated condition.

Dr. C. Requires a Meeting with Her Adult Patient's Parents Who Pay for His Treatment

Clinical vignette: Mr. M. is a 30-year-old gay man who contacts Dr. C. hoping to begin psychotherapy after Mr. M.'s psychotherapist of 9 years retires. Mr. M. is financially supported by his family in California; during his 9 years of treatment, which began after his graduation from college and move to a large East Coast city, Mr. M. has intermittently taken adult education classes and worked on an unfinished autobiographical novel, but has never had paid work. He had understood his psychotherapy as focused primarily on his challenges with dating. During his 9 years of treatment, Mr. M.'s therapist had no contact with his family other than sending to them Mr. M.'s monthly bills for treatment.

Dr. C. completes her evaluation over three sessions, and her diagnostic impression is consistent with mid-level BPO with narcissistic features. As part of the evaluation and because Mr. M.'s treatment has been paid for by his parents, Dr. C. conveys to Mr. M. a wish to meet with Mr. M. and his parents when they are next visiting, which happens to coincide with the completion of their evaluation. Mr. M. reacts with a mix of concern and anger. He explains that his prior treater had considered their psychotherapy "sacred" and had refused to allow contact from Mr. M.'s parents even though they had expressed concern about Mr. M.'s lack of progress toward meaningful work. Dr. C. explains her rationale for the meeting informed by her desire to learn more about Mr. M. from his parents and to educate them about her diagnostic impression and the treatment she is proposing, which includes a requirement for work or school. Mr. M. grudgingly agrees to this meeting while protesting: "My therapist understood that I had to get my romantic life going before I could decide on a career so he kept my parents out of this and you can't seem to appreciate that!"

Take Home Point: The TFP therapist may need to confront directly a patient's omnipotent control expressed as demand to keep the treatment relationship a "closed system."

4.3   The Role of Family Meetings in TFP

> - *TFP clinicians will offer family meetings for many patients in the assessment phase.*
> - *TFP clinicians will almost always require a family meeting in the assessment phase when the family is paying for treatment.*
> - *TFP clinicians will recommend regular follow-up family meetings for certain patients.*
> - *TFP clinicians will offer to help with referrals for family therapy if indicated.*

The family meeting in the TFP assessment phase has multiple goals. This meeting will occur toward the end of the assessment phase, when the clinician has developed a preliminary, but clear, diagnostic impression, prior to the initiation of the contracting phase. The therapist will use the meeting as an opportunity to collect valuable parallel information about the patient as part of this initial phase as would happen frequently in a standard "medical model" assessment. Because some BPO and BPD patients will frequently present extreme, caricatured portraits of the important people in their lives, the meeting with the patient's parents, spouse, or partner can sometimes serve as a useful antidote to those accounts. Adult patients paying for their own treatment understandably will reserve the right to accept or decline a family meeting as part of the assessment. The situation differs somewhat for adult patients who are dependent on others and whose treatment is paid for by parents, siblings, or spouses.

Why would the TFP therapist strongly encourage, if not insist on, a family meeting when assessing the financially dependent patient? TFP's structural interview and assessment process pays particular attention to subtle forms of antisocial activity seen in patients exhibiting parasitism of different kinds. The notion of the parasitic, exploitative personality disordered patient is more clearly delineated in TFP than in the other evidence-based treatments for BPD. When adult patients are financially supported, it is critical that the clinician explores the possibility of passive exploitation, which is a threat to true progress and requires some family involvement in the treatment process.

Many families will want some kind of supportive treatment themselves to help them best manage the challenges of a family member with a severe PD. The TFP therapist will be open to helping the family in this way and will require permission from the patient for coordination with the family's therapist as the treatment proceeds. This kind of adjunctive treatment may be available for families on an individual basis or through family group meetings such as the Family Connections program of the National Educational Alliance for Borderline Personality Disorder or TARA (Treatment and Research Advancements – National Association for Personality Disorders) [11].

Ms. N.'s Therapist Uses a Family Meeting with Her Patient's Parents as Part of the Evaluation Process to Gather History and to Provide Psychoeducation

Clinical vignette: Ms. N. is a 21-year-old woman with BPD. She is enrolled in college but relies heavily on her parents for support, spending all of her weekends with them and dropping in without notice many nights each week. Her parents have attempted without success to set limits on Ms. N.'s intrusion into their daily lives; twice she threatened to jump off their terrace if they stood firm on the limits they wished to impose. When Ms. N.'s parents plan a week's vacation overseas, Ms. N. reacted by taking an overdose requiring an emergency room visit.

When Ms. N. is referred for TFP, her parents ask to meet with her new therapist and outline their concerns

(continued)

(continued)

about Ms. N.'s pattern of dependency. The therapist scheduled a family session that included the patient after the therapist's evaluation sessions and her discussion of her diagnostic impression with the patient. In the family session, the therapist reviewed her diagnostic impression of BPD with a layperson's description of how to understand this condition, explaining the interaction of a predisposition to intense emotional responses interacting with problematic internal representations of self and others. The therapist helped Ms. N.'s parents understand that it was not unreasonable to expect a certain level of behavioral control from their daughter and that her overdose was motivated by multiple reasons that may likely have included the wish to influence their feelings and behavior. The therapist expressed empathy for the conflict they experienced between wanting to limit Ms. N.'s dependence on them and support her autonomous growth on the one hand and their anxiety about her dangerous acting out on the other. As a means of helping them negotiate this conflict, her TFP therapist strongly encourages Ms. N.'s parents to seek consultation with a family therapist with TFP training who might help them manage their anxiety when setting limits. The family therapist meeting with Ms. N.'s parents strongly supports their reasonable expectations for Ms. N.'s conduct. Ms. N.'s therapist and the family therapist continue to communicate regularly to review the progress in both treatments.

Take Home Point: The therapist's involvement with family members can be a critically helpful component of TFP treatment and should be considered as part of the evaluation process for any patient who is dependent in some important way on family support.

4.4   TFP Openness About Diagnosis and Prognosis

- *TFP clinicians will share their diagnostic impressions with families.*
- *TFP clinicians will discuss patients' prognosis with families.*
- *TFP clinicians may need to engage in detailed discussions about the role of co-occurring conditions.*
- *TFP clinicians may need to help families distinguish between certain conditions (depression, anxiety, attention disorders) and personality disorders.*
- *TFP clinicians will engage families in frank discussion about suicide risk.*

TFP therapists will conclude the assessment process with a prospective patient with an open and clear discussion of the therapist's diagnostic impression. This process should include a methodical review of both personality disorder symptoms and symptoms reflecting co-occurring conditions. The prioritization of a frank discussion of personality disorder diagnoses is now the implicit standard of care in all of the evidence-based treatments for BPD [12]. There is less consensus about a comparably frank discussion of narcissistic personality disorder (NPD) traits, and some experts have suggested alternative ways of conveying central elements of the disorder especially given the DSM-5's relatively narrow description focusing on grandiosity and arrogance and many NPD patients' fragility and exquisite sensitivity to perceived criticism [13].

TFP therapists will extend this frank discussion of diagnoses to their work with families. This process should include a detailed discussion of the disorder and its prognosis. The findings from important prospective studies done in recent years support the therapist's ability to convey a relatively good prognosis for BPD, albeit with certain provisos [14, 15].

Similar data is not available for other diagnostic presentations (narcissistic, hypochondriacal, dependent), and the data on the prognosis for antisocial personality disorder (ASPD) remains particularly discouraging [16].

Families are often oriented to better-known and more easily understood diagnostic categories such as mood, anxiety, and attention disorders, which can make initiation of discussion of a personality disorder challenging if not contentious. Often families have been told that a patient has a "treatment-resistant depression" or an "atypical bipolar disorder" diagnosis. In these cases family members may become angry when a new clinician suggests that the symptoms unresponsive to treatment reflect some other diagnosis. This negative response can be exacerbated when a clinician suggests that the diagnosis in question is usually most effectively treated with psychotherapy and not medication. The new clinician may then be the target of misplaced anger toward prior treaters who had emphasized pharmacologic solutions.

On the other hand, some families may welcome a discussion of personality disorder diagnoses, particularly if they have been witness over many years to family members' failure to respond to standard treatments, often with concerning side effects. These families may explore the PD literature on their own or access psychoeducation or support groups. The engaged family can be a critical asset in TFP treatment and in some cases essential to the success of the treatment.

Frank discussion of the suicide risk for patients with BPD and other PDs is another cornerstone of family involvement. The clinician treating a BPD patient with multiple high lethality attempts will need to educate family members about the statistics for completed suicide in BPD (approaching 10 %) and the limitation on prediction and prevention across treatment modalities [17]. Such family psychoeducation is consistent with the TFP principle of taking whatever steps are required to assist the therapist in feeling as safe as possible. The therapist who has been able to meet with the family of a patient with serious, recurrent suicidality and has therefore been able to document the content of this meeting has "gone the extra mile" in self-protection.

Ms. O.'s Father Is Concerned that Her Therapist's TFP
Approach Is Insufficiently Supportive

Clinical vignette: Ms. O. is a divorced woman in her early 40s who is referred to Ms. D., a social worker therapist with TFP training, after her psychiatrist of 15 years moves away. Ms. O. is under the impression that she suffers from "treatment-resistant depression, panic attacks, and attention deficit disorder." When Ms. O. first meets with Ms. D., she is in a crisis as she only recently broke off a romantic relationship and is actively suicidal with thoughts of jumping from the roof of her office building. Ms. O. works part-time in a low-paying position despite her training as an accountant, and her treatment is paid for by her father.

Ms. D. meets initially with Ms. O. and learns from an extended evaluation that Ms. O. has had lifelong marked rejection sensitivity, long-standing suicidal thinking, and intermittent non-suicidal self-injurious behavior including head banging and burning herself with a cigarette on her torso when she is experiencing marked distress. Ms. O. reports she frequently spoke with her psychiatrist while in crisis in the evening and on weekends and was able to call him at his home "whenever I needed his help."

After the evaluation process is completed, Ms. D. feels she has enough information to discuss with Ms. O. her diagnostic impression that includes a primary personality disorder with borderline traits and possible co-occurring conditions including mood and anxiety disorders. She introduces Ms. O. to the essential elements of TFP including the therapist's limitations on crisis management between sessions and the patient's responsibility for staying safe or using local emergency department services if necessary. The following day she hears from Ms.

(continued)

(continued)

O.'s father; he is alarmed at the apparent change in diagnostic thinking and the limits on contact given his sense that Ms. O.'s prior psychiatrist "kept her alive" by his availability.

Ms. D. recommends a meeting with Ms. O. and her father. She explains her diagnostic thinking and suggests that Ms. O.'s personality disorder symptoms have contributed to her limited capacity for work and explains why 15 years of proactive pharmacothearpy with the newest antidepressants available was ineffective. Ms. O.'s father is open to the change in thinking about diagnosis, but he and Ms. O. protest what they experience as a negligent and withholding approach related to availability for support between sessions. Ms. D. feels under attack with Ms. O. and her father in the room both appearing angry, but she methodically returns to the TFP treatment contract and explains why she feels frequent contacts and limitless availability may have hindered Ms. O.'s recovery. Ms. D. goes to lengths during a second meeting with Ms. O. and her father to explain the differences between depression symptoms and affective instability; she also makes a point of reviewing the relative limitations of medication treatment for personality disorders and the likely need for a psychotherapy developed specifically for the disorder to replace the long-standing, gratifying, but limitedly effective treatment she had been receiving with her prior treater. Ms. O. and her father remain concerned, but Ms. O. agrees to move forward with treatment under the terms Ms. D. has outlined.

Take Home Point: The TFP therapist will strongly encourage family involvement, which can include psychoeducation about diagnosis and prognosis and explanation of the TFP approach.

4.5   Discussion About the Particulars of TFP and Treatment-Interfering Behaviors

- *Families may find TFP's approach uncomfortably different from patients' prior treatments or may welcome its new perspective.*
- *Families may be disturbed by TFP's management of suicidality or may find it addresses a burden they have been carrying.*
- *Families may not agree with TFP's approach to treatment-interfering behaviors or may see it as reasonable and useful.*
- *Families may find TFP's requirement for meaningful work or school to be unrealistic or unfair – or may find it a relief from the idea that their loved one is condemned to a life of nonfunctioning or dependency.*

For many families the overarching theory of TFP and the specifics of the TFP assessment process, contracting phase, and details of ongoing TFP treatment will be novel if not counterintuitive. Families familiar with some clinician's practice of pharmacotherapy, supportive psychotherapy, or dialectical behavior therapy (DBT) for personality disorder symptoms may find TFP overly confrontational or insufficiently sympathetic toward the patient. The TFP clinician will often need to explain in detail a number of the elements of the treatment to family members and to hold firm to the central tenets of the treatment even if met with pushback by families. As is the case when establishing the treatment contract (the basic tenets of the therapy) with the patient, if there is a major disagreement regarding some of the central understandings of the treatment approach, it may not be best to move forward with the treatment. However, if the patient expresses genuine interest in the therapy, it is generally best to move forward even if the parents have some reservations, with the plan for follow-up meetings with the patient and parents as the therapy progresses.

Because many PD patients will present for treatment in distress, families may be confused by the TFP approach which begins with a two- or three-session evaluation followed by a contracting phase that requires at least two sessions and can extend to many more. The anxious family concerned about the patient's difficulties may expect "therapy" to begin immediately and may need help in understanding the logic behind the TFP assessment and contracting process.

It is easy to imagine a family member's concern or even outrage at various junctures in the TFP process preceding the beginning of the treatment. Many patients may never have been told their diagnoses, so learning of the therapist's impression of a likely personality disorder may come as a surprise. Families may be confused to learn that the primary intervention for a PD diagnosis is psychotherapy, not medication, particularly when prior treaters may have emphasized the commonly co-occurring conditions (dysphoria, anxiety) and conveyed an expectation that medication would address those symptoms effectively.

Families are often particularly confused by the TFP approach to suicidality. Many families feel that the "always available" therapist willing to field calls from the suicidal patient on nights and weekends or visit the suicidal patient in the emergency room or inpatient psychiatric unit is highly likely to be of help to the patient. The TFP therapist is therefore obliged to explain why setting limits on contact between sessions for suicidal "emergencies" or minimizing the "secondary gain" of extra sessions or the therapist's interceding in other treatment settings would be in the patient's long-term interest. In a typical scenario, a concerned parent may contact the therapist early in the TFP contracting phase exclaiming: "Our daughter says she wouldn't be able to call you if she were suicidal! How would this help her?" Patients can recruit families to share their powerfully held beliefs about the uncaring clinician ignoring the suffering patient; only the clinician's clear, considered explanation of TFP's approach in advance can help avoid certain situations of families joining the patient in an accusation of abandonment. In these situations, it is important to be clear that the patient and family have the choice of a more overtly supportive therapy that may do less to improve the patient's autonomous functioning or TFP, which includes that as a major goal.

The TFP contracting phase will include the expectation that the patient will be engaged in meaningful work or studies as part of the treatment. This expectation may seem unfair to some families who have been convinced by patients (often with support from prior treaters) that the patient is too impaired to participate in meaningful activity. The family may feel that this requirement is presumptuous, reflecting the therapist's inadequate understanding of the patient's disability. Here the TFP therapist might suggest that based on experience it is often the case that BPD patients often can do more than they imagine. The therapist will also point out how engagement in activity may be challenging but also therapeutic. Families may emphasize the patient's co-occurring medical or psychiatric conditions in which case the therapist would outline the steps required to first address those conditions and question any resistance to doing so as possibly reflecting the patient's continued wish to opt for a passive role in life and be provided for by the family or by the government or insurance disability payments. The therapist will underscore it is ultimately the patient who should decide if TFP, with its requirements for work or studies, is, in fact, the right treatment.

Mr. F.'s Family Is Alarmed by His Therapist's Approach to Intersession Availability

Clinical vignette: Mr. F. is a 45-year-old married man who had been in a supportive psychotherapy for over 10 years when his therapist died suddenly. Mr. F. considered his therapist to be a central figure of support during those 10 years which were marked by the gradual dissolution

(continued)

(continued)

of Mr. F.'s marriage, a deteriorating performance at work, and intermittent threats of self-harm. Mr. F. described himself as "at a loss" after this therapist's death; he reluctantly agreed to meet with Dr. G. for an evaluation, as he was recommended to Mr. F. as a talented diagnostician with a good reputation.

Mr. F. was immediately put off by Dr. G., particularly Dr. G.'s discussion of personality disorder symptoms (Mr. F. had understood his condition to be "atypical bipolar depression") and Dr. G.'s policy of not being available between sessions (Mr. F.'s previous therapist had been easily accessible for support evenings and weekends when Mr. F. felt suicidal). Mr. F. was also confused by Dr. G.'s recommendation that he meet with Mr. F.'s wife and sister who were helping to pay his therapy bills.

At the outset of the meeting with Dr. G., Mr. F.'s sister expressed her concern about the stated policy on contact between sessions. She had often heard her brother talk of the solace he received from his emergency calls to his deceased therapist and wondered why Dr. G. would not provide similar help. Dr. G. used the family meeting to explain at length his TFP approach and to suggest that the availability of the therapist may have undermined Mr. F.'s ability to assume responsibility for controlling his impulses and managing his affects. He conveyed that he thought Mr. F. was able to control his suicidal feelings between sessions and outlined the plan (emergency room evaluation, possible inpatient hospitalization) should that not be possible. Mr. F.'s family remained wary of this new approach but agreed that the treatment during the preceding years had not seemed to help Mr. F. in critical aspects of his functioning.

Take Home Point: The TFP therapist may need to meet with family members to explain the rationale behind certain elements of the treatment to allay family members' concerns.

4.6   Family Support in Addressing Patient's Omnipotent Control

- *The TFP approach assumes most PD patients are capable of controlling self-destructive behaviors to a large extent and will convey this expectation to families.*
- *The TFP approach assumes most PD patients are able to engage in some kind or meaningful activity (work or school) and will convey this expectation to families.*
- *The TFP therapist will directly address secondary gain through unhealthy dependency on families.*
- *In extreme cases the therapist will focus on protecting family members from the patient's exploitation.*

TFP is an individual psychotherapy predicated on a patient's desire to make changes toward improved functioning. The treatment is anchored by the therapist's and patient's understanding of the patient's specific goals, not simply a wish to "know myself better" or "get the support I need" but to make actual changes in the major spheres of work and relationships. Elucidation of these goals can sometimes require extended exploration, as many PD patients will focus initially on perceived impairments or limitations and reveal wishes for change only with time.

The TFP therapist will consider the following: Can I engage this patient in the process of identifying personal goals and structure a treatment with this aim in mind? Or, is this patient not genuinely interested in opportunities to move forward, in which case is a referral to case management or a more custodial care recommended?

In the vast majority of cases, the TFP therapist is faced with a highly ambivalent patient and a confused and conflicted family. The therapist will often identify the patient's use of omnipotent control in the family dynamic, for example, the patient insisting on unquestioningly supportive and generous parents or spouse (maintaining the idealized "good object") and alternating with accusations and threats when parents or spouse convey expectations or realistic limits to their support (dominating and controlling the feared "bad object").

If the TFP therapist assesses the patient to have the required minimum health-seeking personality traits allowing the treatment to go forward, the therapist's next step would be to offer the family psychoeducation. Take, for example, the family overwhelmed by a son's recurrent suicidal threats or gestures. One alternative would be to recommend cognitive-behavioral or DBT to help the patient manage these self-destructive impulses. Another possibility would be to offer the patient TFP and to engage the family in discussion of the patient's controlling behaviors, inviting them to establish their own "frame" in tandem with the TFP contracting and frame process. (In this case, the patient who had previously insisted his parents leave work emergently to care for him when he was suicidal would understand that his parents would no longer respond in this manner, after they had put into place an alternative approach to these episodes.)

TFP also addresses directly patients' insistence that they are too ill to engage in meaningful studies or work. Again, parents and spouses will often need psychoeducation and support to move from a stance of resignation to one of informed confrontation. The TFP therapist can expect some families to react negatively to this position. Unfortunately there are cases when the TFP therapist's effectiveness will be directly undermined by families and spouses unwilling or unable to set limits on patients resistant to meeting the work or school requirement. Family dynamics are complicated and can include "system's" reasons to perpetuate a patient's dependency.

In rare cases the therapist will conclude, generally in cases where the patient has very strong antisocial features, that the patient's destructive impulses are so powerful as to preclude meaningful treatment of any kind. In these cases patients are often so embracing of the "sick role," expressed through self-destructive behaviors or somatic preoccupations, as to render exploratory psychotherapy of any kind useless. In these cases the therapist's role is sometimes reduced to protecting family members from the patient's unchecked destructive impulses. One common story is the patient with low BPO with borderline and narcissistic traits whose symptoms evolve over time from primarily psychiatric (depression, anxiety) to primarily somatic. Patients embracing somatic symptoms can sometimes incur tremendous medical costs, expecting family members to pay these bills given the patients' sense of themselves as incapacitated. In these cases the therapist's attention might be focused on helping the family protect themselves from inordinate sacrifices or expenses, understood by the therapist as the patient's expression of omnipotent control maintaining an idealized, nurturing other.

Ms. Y.'s Husband Shares Her Conviction that She Is Incapable of Meaningful Activity

Clinical vignette: Ms. Y. is a 30-year-old separated woman, supported entirely by her estranged husband. Ms. Y. has been hospitalized twice for suicidal threats in the past year in the context of her conflictual marital relationship. Ms. Y. spends most of her time watching television or shopping; she has not worked outside the home since her marriage 7 years ago.

Dr. E. sees Ms. Y. in consultation for TFP; Ms. Y. articulates her goals as "feeling better about myself, having a better sense of my goals and values, and developing some type of career, maybe in the arts." Dr. E. meets with Ms. Y. and her husband and outlines the TFP contract which includes the expectation that the patient works or engages in meaningful studies. Both Ms. Y. and her

(continued)

(continued)

husband balk at this proposal, feeling that her recent hospitalizations and recurrent suicidality reflect an intractable fragility making work or school impossible.

Dr. E. explains to Mr. Y., as he had individually with Ms. Y., that he understands that engaging in a structured activity with other people will be stressful and arouse anxiety in Ms. Y. He goes on to explain that the two weekly therapy sessions provide the opportunity for Ms. Y. to explore the nature of the anxieties that arise in the work setting and that, in the large majority of cases, working on these issues in therapy helps the patient tolerate and adapt to the work setting. With this explanation, the couple decides to accept Dr. E.'s recommendations.

Take Home Point: The TFP therapist may need to meet with family members to explain the TFP requirement for meaningful work or studies when the patient has convinced family members such activity is either harmful or not possible.

4.7   Family Involvement in Pharmacotherapy

- *Families should be aware of the limited, adjunctive role of medications in the treatment of personality disorder symptoms.*
- *Families should be aware of the active goal of reducing most medication regimens.*
- *Families should be aware of the serious side effects of many medications, including risk in overdose.*
- *TFP clinicians may need to educate families about the psychodynamic meanings of medication use for patients.*

Most family members are surprised to learn that medications are considered adjunctive, at best, for the treatment of personality disorder symptoms. PD diagnoses are rarely made in adolescence (although emerging data suggests they can and should be made in certain cases), and many patients will have PD symptoms for years, if not decades, before a diagnosis is made and conveyed to the patient and family [18].

Therefore, in this intervening period, many family members have come to expect that medications for mood, anxiety, attention, or sleep disorders would effectively address the constellation of PD symptoms they observe. Clinicians will often accentuate the diagnoses co-occurring with personality disorders and will minimize or dismiss the contribution of PD symptoms to a clinical picture. Also, clinicians will rarely educate families about the critical point that the patient with, for example, a personality disorder like BPD and a major depressive disorder will not respond as robustly to standard treatments for depression as would the patient with the depressive disorder alone.

The TFP therapist will be "swimming against the tide" by, first, underscoring the centrality of the PD symptoms and, second, advocating for the most limited medication regimen possible for the patient in treatment. This approach requires the TFP therapist to consider the meaning for the patient of continued polypharmacy and the likely response to a recommendation for a more restricted regimen. Patients will often experience this recommendation as punitive or withholding, convincing family members that they are being "deprived" of the relief they associate with the act of receiving medications.

It is important that patients and families become fully educated about the real risks associated with many of the medications commonly prescribed for patients with PDs and co-occurring conditions. Families should be aware, for example, that lithium carbonate and tricyclic antidepressants are toxic in overdose, that benzodiazepines are potentially habit forming, that non-compliance with an MAOI diet leads to serious complications including death, and that widely used atypical antipsychotic medications are associated with metabolic syndrome including obesity. Because prescribers often find themselves reacting to PD patients in crisis by adding medications ad hoc, many PD patients wind up on complicated, unwieldy combinations.

For the TFP therapist who cannot prescribe, these complex circumstances require the therapist to have an active, engaged relationship with the prescriber. The TFP therapist may need to act as go-between, mediating between the family and prescriber, to insure the family is adequately educated about the role of medications and their risks.

The TFP therapist will develop an understanding about the meaning of medication for a particular patient. A common scenario is the passive patient who wants medication to "do the work" freeing the patient from the requirement for effort or motivation, often leading the patient to fault the prescriber and medications along the lines of "They can't seem to get the right medications for me." Another pattern might be the patient who suffers persistently with unpleasant side effects like obesity, hypersomnia, or lowered libido, confirming an experience of the prescriber as hurtful and callous. The therapist appreciating these object relations will therefore be inclined to address these patterns with the patient and family.

Ms. D. and Her Spouse Worry that a Medication Taper Will Be "Depriving"

Clinical vignette: Ms. D. is a married woman who comes to Dr. L. for a consultation after a suicide attempt by overdose following the discovery of her husband's infidelity. Ms. D. has been seen by a psychiatrist monthly for 5 years; she is prescribed a stimulant, antidepressant, and benzodiazepine. Dr. L. feels comfortable sharing with Ms. D. her diagnostic impression which includes a mid- to high BPO with circumscribed borderline traits which tend to surface in times of stress.

(continued)

(continued)

Dr. L. meets with Ms. D. and her husband. Dr. L. initiates a discussion of her goal to taper Ms. D.'s medication regimen as tolerated. Dr. L. has concerns that Ms. D.'s use of stimulants may have caused her difficulties and feels Ms. D.'s stated indication for continued use of stimulants – to help her stay awake and drive more carefully when going to her beach house on weekends – is not an appropriate use of the medication. Ms. D. and her husband are initially concerned that Dr. L. is "taking away" a medication helpful, in its way, in the past. Dr. L. feels comfortable outlining for Ms. D. and her husband a hypothesis that being given medication she may not require nevertheless has felt gratifying, particularly as she had felt her husband was pulling away in recent months. Dr. L. feels more comfortable paring Ms. D.'s regimen after the family meeting having preemptively addressed a potential "split" that might have made the goal of decreasing medications more difficult.

Take Home Point: Meeting with a patient and family member to provide information about the limits of pharmacotherapy in the treatment of personality disorder symptoms can help the prescriber address a potential "split" in a proactive way.

4.8 Family Involvement and Risk Management

- Family involvement is a cornerstone of effective risk management for clinicians treating PD patients.
- TFP's openness to family involvement can limit splitting.
- TFP's active addressing of patient's omnipotent control can limit families' displaced anger.

The risk management literature underscores central tenets for clinician self-protection particularly important in the treatment of patients with severe personality disorders [19]. One central risk management adage stresses that angry family members are sometimes a critical element in malpractice suits, often but not always in cases of completed suicide, among other scenarios [20]. It is easy to imagine how the commonly described reasons for litigation in psychiatry, such as suicide, medication side effects, privacy violations, and boundary crossings, could be complicated by PD diagnoses.

Family involvement as described in TFP is both good treatment and good risk management. Because TFP strongly endorses family involvement as part of the assessment process, the potential for a future "split" is significantly diminished at the start of treatment. In TFP for BPD, the family meeting will address the real risk of completed suicide, particularly for those patients with histories of recurrent suicide gestures or attempts. In certain cases the TFP therapist will soberly convey that treatment is no guarantee of any particular outcome despite the family's and therapist's best intentions.

TFP's active family involvement preemptively addresses the common pitfall of the frustrated and anxious family feeling powerless about expressing their concerns to a family member's treater. A PD patient might be motivated to keep the treater and family apart, controlling the information each party receives. This dynamic can be explosive should there be some kind of untoward event, leading to a family's recriminatory response, possibly with legal action.

Ms. P.'s Parents Are Kept in the Dark About Her Treatment

Clinical vignette: Ms. P. is a graduate student with BPD marked by multiple suicide gestures and attempts. Her parents follow a recommendation to send her to a

(continued)

long-term residential treatment facility at great expense. Ms. P.'s therapist at this facility has a policy of not communicating with patients' families, feeling this risks undermining the patient's trust. Ms. P.'s family grows increasingly concerned about her behavior at the facility, which includes persistent alcohol and drug abuse and occasional self-injury by cutting. While Ms. P.'s parents are in contact with the facility's director, they are rebuffed when reaching out to the therapist after a particularly concerning incident.

Soon after this incident, Ms. P.'s parents are contacted by the residential facility late one night after Ms. P. is hospitalized emergently following an overdose of benzodiazepines prescribed by the program's psychiatrist. At some point when Ms. P. is still on the hospital's intensive care unit, her father, an attorney, calls Ms. P.'s therapist and the facility director and warns that he will take legal action against them should Ms. P. die from her overdose.

After Ms. P. recovers from his overdose, her parents insist she return home and seek treatment as an outpatient locally. Her new therapist using a TFP approach insists on family involvement at the outset, despite Ms. P.'s initial resistance. The TFP therapist outlines her requirement for ongoing family involvement and relative transparency about some, but not all, elements of the treatment for Ms. P. going forward. Over time Ms. P.'s parents' attitude shifts from confrontational to collaborative with this different approach.

Take Home Point: Family involvement is an essential part of a good risk management approach for clinicians treating patients with severe personality disorder pathology.

References

1. Clarkin JF, Yeomans FE, Kernberg OF. Transference-focused psychotherapy for borderline personality disorder: a clinical guide. 1st ed. Arlington, VA: American Psychiatric Publishing; 2014.
2. Hoffman PD, Fruzzetti AE. Advances in interventions for families with a relative with a personality disorder diagnosis. Cur Psychiatr Rep. 2007;9:68–73.
3. Linehan MM. Cognitive-behavioral treatment of borderline personality disorder. New York: Guilford Press; 1993.
4. Bateman AW, Fonagy P. Mentalization-based therapy for borderline personality disorder: a practical guide. New York: Oxford University Press; 2006.
5. Young JE, Klosko JS, Weisharr ME. Schema therapy: a practitioner's guide. New York: Guilford Press; 2003.
6. Silk KR. Augmenting psychotherapy for borderline personality disorder: the STEPPS program. Am J Psychiatr. 2008;165(4):413–5.
7. Silk KR, Feurino L. Psychopharmacology of personality disorder. In: Widiger TA, editor. The Oxford handbook of personality disorders. New York: Oxford University Press; 2012. p. 713–26.
8. Gunderson JG, Links P. Handbook of good psychiatric management for borderline personality disorder. Arlington, VA: American Psychiatric Publishing; 2014.
9. Porr V. Overcoming borderline personality disorder: a family guide for healing and change. New York: Oxford University Press; 2010.
10. Gunderson JG, Hoffman PD. Understanding and treating borderline personality disorder: a guide for professionals and families. Arlington, VA: American Psychiatric Publishing; 2005.
11. Hoffman PD, Fruzzetti AE, Buteau E, Neiditch ER, Penney D, Bruce ML, et al. Family connections: a program for relatives of persons with borderline personality disorder. Fam Process. 2005;44(2):217–25.
12. Weinberg I, Ronningstam E, Goldblatt MJ, Schecter M, Maltsberger JT. Common factors in empirically supported treatments of borderline personality disorder. Curr Psychiatr Rep. 2011;13:60–8.

13. Caligor E, Clarkin JF, Kernberg OF. Handbook of dynamic psychotherapy for higher level personality pathology. Washington, DC: American Psychiatric Press; 2007.
14. Zanarini MC, Frankenburg FR, Reich DB, Fitzmaurice G. Attainment and stability of sustained symptomatic remission and recovery among patients with borderline personality disorder and axis II comparison subjects: a 16-year prospective follow-up study. Am J Psychiatr. 2012;169(5):476–83.
15. Gunderson JG, Stout RL, McGlashan TH, Shea MT, Morey LC, Grilo CM, et al. Ten-year course of borderline personality. Arch Gen Psychiatr. 2011;68(8):827–37.
16. Black DW, Baumgard CH, Bell SE. The long-term outcome of antisocial personality disorder compared with depression, schizophrenia and surgical conditions. Bull Am Acad Psychiatr Law. 1995;23(1):43–52.
17. Goodman M, Roiff T, Oakes AH, Paris J. Suicidal risk and management in borderline personality disorder. Curr Psychiatr Rep. 2012;14(1):79–85.
18. Chanen A, McCutcheon L. Prevention and early intervention for borderline personality disorder: current status and recent evidence. Br J Psychiatr. 2013;202(s54):s24–9.
19. Gutheil TG. Medicolegal pitfalls in the treatment of borderline patients. Am J Psychiatr. 1985;142:9–14.
20. Gutheil TG. Suicide, suicide litigation, and borderline personality disorder. J Pers Disord. 2004;18:248–56.

Chapter 5
Transference-Focused Psychotherapy (TFP) Principles in Inpatient Psychiatry

1. *TFP principles can provide clinicians with an overarching approach to the psychiatric hospitalization of patients with significant personality disorder pathology.*
2. *The TFP contract explores, in advance, contingencies related to psychiatric hospitalization.*
3. *TFP principles can be of use to clinicians evaluating the risks and benefits of psychiatric hospitalization, even if the clinicians involved do not have a clearly established relationship with the patient.*
4. *TFP principles can aid outpatient and inpatient clinicians in minimizing the risks associated with hospitalization.*
5. *TFP principles can aid outpatient and inpatient clinicians in maximizing the benefits associated with hospitalization.*

5.1 Introduction

The role of inpatient psychiatric hospitalization in the treatment of patients with serious personality disorder (PD) pathology remains critical despite the significant changes in practice patterns in recent decades [1]. The era of the extended inpatient

© Springer International Publishing Switzerland 2016
R.G. Hersh et al., *Fundamentals of Transference-Focused Psychotherapy*,
DOI 10.1007/978-3-319-44091-0_5

psychiatric hospitalization for patients with a primary personality disorder diagnosis, made famous by the book and movie *Girl, Interrupted*, is over in the United States for all but the very few who can afford it. Instead, psychiatric hospitalizations for patients with PD symptoms are usually relatively brief – days to weeks rather than months to years. Currently, hospitalization for patients with PDs can serve to: (1) provide relative safety at a time of high risk, (2) refine diagnostic understanding, (3) review a patient's medication regimen, and (4) reassess the overarching treatment plan.

The psychiatric hospitalization of a patient with significant personality disorder pathology in current times is invariably fraught, often occurring during a period of heightened affect for both the patient and the responsible clinician. Elective psychiatric hospitalizations, planned weeks in advance, are rare. For a psychiatric hospitalization to be approved by many payers, the patient's condition must be demonstrably deteriorating. These situations can include: episodes marked by emerging frank psychosis; escalating suicidal thoughts, feelings, or actions; severe adverse medication reactions; grave substance use or eating disorder symptoms; or some combination of this list.

Because the process of assessing a PD patient for hospitalization is inevitably done in an atmosphere of anxiety for both treaters and patients and families, it is easy for a clinician to become overwhelmed, confused, or even panicked. Families and patients, too, may be fearful, if not frankly paranoid, about a prospective psychiatric hospitalization; alternatively, patients and families may anticipate a magical cure for what has become an overwhelming or exhausting situation or perhaps harbor a pleasant fantasy about a "rest cure"-like retreat, no longer the reality of today's high-turnover inpatient psychiatry services. All such attitudes are likely challenging to clinicians. TFP principles may offer clinicians a systematic way to approach the decision-making about hospitalization and patient management during hospitalization, using both psychodynamic thinking about transference and countertransference currents and information about the risks and benefits of psychiatric hospitalization that have accrued over the years and been refined by experts on the subject [2, 3].

In the TFP contracting process, as part of an individual outpatient therapy, the therapist and patient together will explore the various contingencies related to inpatient hospitalization. It is easy to imagine the variety and complexity of these contingencies, given the many possible clinical situations that can arise and the likely divergent motivations and attitudes of those who might be involved. The questions the therapist and patient will need to explore in advance include: Who initiates a hospitalization? For what possible reasons? With what goals? At what kind of facility? Who makes the final determination about hospitalization? In many cases there are multiple parties involved: patient, therapist, other clinicians (as in a split treatment), family, and payers, among others. It is important to remember that a psychiatric hospitalization might be related directly to a patient's PD symptoms (suicidality, homicidality, impulsivity), but may also be indicated because of heightened acuity related to a co-occurring condition (depression, substance use, eating disorder).

It may also be useful to consider ways that TFP principles can aid clinicians in roles other than primary therapist. These principles may be helpful to clinicians working on psychiatric inpatient units, informing their approach and increasing the likelihood that hospitalization benefits will outweigh risks. In addition, this chapter will extend the use of TFP principles to those clinicians in outpatient programs (partial hospital, intensive outpatient), consultation-liaison services, and emergency rooms, often involved in this process of hospitalizing PD patients. In these cases, clinicians may find themselves assuming a critical role in the hospitalization process without primary responsibility for the patient's care, with a limited history with the patient, often reliant on incomplete information, and functioning in a period of heightened affect.

The risks associated with hospitalization for the patient with BPD are many and well-described [4]. They include:

regression in the hospital environment; loss of the structure of work or school; the influence of exposure to other patients' destructive or self-destructive behaviors; and resultant poly-pharmacy, often of limited value with unintended, negative consequences. While the TFP therapist will commit to a degree of involvement when a patient is hospitalized, the involvement has clear limits, and the goals of involvement are circumscribed. As noted, the TFP therapist's ambition, if possible, is to have the patient return to individual treatment and to have potentially treatment-interfering behaviors addressed in the treatment process. The hospitalization therefore can present risks of introducing or exacerbating treatment-interfering behaviors: for example, the employed patient who loses a job because of a hospitalization or the patient begun on sedating antipsychotic medication causing attendance at school to be compromised. These treatment-interfering behaviors may be inadvertently supported by the inpatient team, making the outpatient TFP clinician's role one involving education and delicate negotiation. While splits between outpatient and inpatient clinicians have often been observed as part of the hospitalization of patients with severe personality pathology, much too has been written about the risks for destructive splitting within inpatient teams when treating certain PD patients [5].

How can the clinicians involved maximize the benefits for the hospitalized patient? The TFP contract focuses on those goals required to have the patient return to therapy or to clarify if, in fact, TFP is the most appropriate treatment. The hospitalization might also provide the opportunity for the therapist to have a session with the patient that addresses deep issues that were difficult to begin to explore in an outpatient office. What can be done during a hospitalization to achieve those goals? The outpatient TFP therapist working in concert with the inpatient team, aware of the risk of splitting between treaters, can aim to insure the hospitalization proves useful for the patient. Even when there is not an outpatient TFP therapist involved, inpatient clinicians may use TFP principles themselves to guide management of hospitalized

PD patients, even if those patients have not had nor are going to be discharged to TFP treatment. These principles for productive use of the hospital setting are closely aligned with the guidelines established by PD experts – experts identified with specific evidence-based treatments as well as those with more eclectic orientations [6].

5.2   TFP Principles Can Provide Clinicians with an Overarching Approach to the Psychiatric Hospitalization of Patients with Significant Personality Disorder Pathology

- *TFP principles, informed by object relations theory, are applicable to certain essential issues associated with hospitalization.*
- *The TFP approach suggests simultaneous openness to benefits and wariness of risks with hospitalization.*
- *The TFP individual therapist will apply central tenets of the treatment to the clinical questions associated with hospitalization.*
- *Treaters without a long-term relationship with the patient can use TFP principles in decision-making about hospitalization.*
- *Inpatient clinicians can use TFP principles in their management of PD patients.*

TFP as an individual psychotherapy provides treaters with a way of thinking about many critical aspects of psychiatric hospitalization. In TFP, the subject of psychiatric hospitalization is explored in the assessment phase, if indicated, and then in the contracting phase, with a thorough discussion of the respective responsibilities of both the patient and therapist should the possibility of hospitalization arise. The TFP contract will describe, in advance, the therapist's attitude toward an involvement in a possible hospitalization so as not to set up a "surprise" for patients and families in the future [7].

What does it mean to have an "object relations-informed" understanding of the psychiatric hospitalization of the patient with PD symptoms? The TFP therapist begins by assessing the patient's level of organization, asking: What is the nature of the patient's identify formation, what are the predominant defensive operations used, and what is the patient's capacity for reality testing? Beyond this, the therapist achieves a sense of the principle object relations dyads (internal sense of self and other) that determine his experience of himself in the world. For example, does the patient tend to experience himself as a victim of others' abuse, as the sensitive person who sees things more clearly than others, or as a competitor with others for control, among other possibilities? The TFP therapist will attempt to understand the implications of a psychiatric hospitalization in this context. The TFP therapist always has in mind the dominant object relations dyad (and its inverse) in play, including with respect to a hospitalization.

The TFP therapist will be at once open to the benefits of hospitalization and concerned about the associated risks. This approach directly addresses the risk of a patient's reflexive idealization or devaluation of a hospitalization. Both are familiar patterns: the patient who imagines the hospital will be a purely supportive, benign environment staffed by caring clinicians or the patient who imagines the hospital as an exclusively punitive, humiliating situation with sadistic doctors and nurses. The TFP therapist will try to avoid suggesting a psychiatric hospitalization as a way to diffuse difficult aspects of the transference (i.e., as a way to diminish or deflect the intensity of the affects emerging in the therapy sessions). The therapist will not offer up the hospitalization as an idealized escape/retreat for the patient, free from any obligations or challenges. The therapist will explain possible benefits from a hospitalization. In his/her decision about hospitalization, the therapist should reflect on his/her reasons to be sure he/she is not recommending hospitalization as part of a countertransference enactment, meaning an action on the therapist's part in response to feelings engendered by the patient that involves acting out one of the patient's internal scenarios rather than observing and exploring it – e.g., hospitalization as saving the patient or punishing the patient or as a way of avoiding emotions that are emerging in the session. In the long run, countertransference enactments undermine the goals of the treatment. The TFP therapist must "keep a foot in reality" when negotiating with a patient wary about hospitalization by outlining how a hospitalization could be of use while also exploring, in the transference, any other meaning the patient might attribute to the decision to hospitalize, such as the idea that the therapist is recommending something the patient perceives to be harmful.

While a primary therapist is usually involved in decision-making about hospitalization, other clinicians in different capacities may also be key figures in this process. For clinicians in consultation-liaison, intensive outpatient or partial hospital, and emergency department roles, assessment of the need for hospitalization is often made with limited information or without a clear treatment alliance. TFP principles used by psychiatry residents in acute care settings may be applicable for more senior clinicians in these situations when the central question relates to psychiatric hospitalization [8, 9]. While some questions related to hospitalization will not necessarily benefit from application of a psychodynamic approach, many will, including the meaning of hospitalization in the context of the patient's individual therapy and as it relates to the patient's relationships with partners and families. The TFP stepwise approach, beginning with diagnostic assessment, even with limited information, and then identification of dominant object relations dyads and their inverses, followed by empathic interventions aimed at putting into words the patient's experience, can be useful even if the clinician will not have a long-standing relationship with the patient.

The inpatient clinician in current times is in a role buffeted by multiple forces. Payers want hospitalizations kept short, while concerns about liability are pressing, given the patients' relatively high level of acuity. Outpatient clinicians may have unreasonable expectations for the results of a hospitalization.

Patients and families may want "therapy" and services not available in the present day or may devalue the kind of treatments that are available. In the setting of these limitations and challenges, inpatient clinicians too can benefit from some of TFP's central tenets: clarity about diagnosis, comfort with discussing PD diagnoses with patients, and identification of critical dyads and their inverses.

Dr. L. Sets a Limit on Mr. B.'s Use of Psychiatric Hospitalization as a Form of Protest

Clinical vignette: Dr. L. is a psychologist treating Mr. B., a patient with an extensive history of substance use (cannabis and alcohol) now in remission for 9 months and borderline personality organization with prominent narcissistic and antisocial traits. Mr. B. is supported by his parents, who have become exhausted over time as Mr. B. has developed a series of excuses for not working, often related to seemingly untreatable somatic complaints.

Dr. L. agrees to work with Mr. B., and while she has significant concerns about his ability to fulfill his responsibilities in their treatment, he reports he is readily willing to do so. Mr. B. takes a low-level job in a copy shop as part of their agreement, complaining bitterly about his co-workers and expressing concern that chemicals from the copy machines are causing him to have daily migraine headaches.

Approximately 2 months into the treatment, Mr. B. leaves a message for Dr. L. letting her know that he will be missing their next appointment, as he feels he has developed "acute depression" related to his work at the copy shop. When Dr. L. calls Mr. B., he angrily consents to come in the following day. At that appointment Mr. B. tells Dr. L. he has been calling the local hospital to see if the psychiatric unit there has an available bed, as he expects he will become suicidal should he go to work the following day and will therefore require rehospitalization.

(continued)

(continued)

Dr. L. had outlined with Mr. B. the contract stipulations related to psychiatric hospitalization and immediately raises her concern that Mr. B.'s motivation for hospitalization may be a response to the initiation of their treatment and a testing of her resolve to keep to their agreement. Mr. B. does not directly answer Dr. L., but repeats that going to the copy shop would be intolerable. Dr. L. suggests to Mr. B. that going to the hospital now would be an action conveying his protest about their treatment, and she encourages him to continue to use their sessions to explore his emerging experience of her as a harsh taskmaster who insists he continue working at a job that will destroy him.

When Mr. B. does not come to his next appointment, Dr. L. calls him at home. She reaches Mr. B.'s brother who reports that Mr. B. is clearly intoxicated and threatening suicide. Dr. L. calls for emergency services to come to Mr. B.'s home; he is admitted first to the emergency department for observation for possible acute alcohol poisoning and then to the psychiatric unit.

Dr. L. arranges a meeting with Mr. B. and his parents while Mr. B. is in the hospital. She again reviews their treatment contract and discusses the options for Mr. B., including return to treatment with her. Mr. B. agrees to come back to treatment with Dr. L. with a plan to go back to work at the copy shop while actively looking for another position that would fulfill his responsibility for work. Dr. L. revisits the topic of hospitalization, reiterating her view that an elective hospitalization as a form of protest is not likely of use to Mr. B., but that an emergent hospitalization, as had just occurred, was required to insure his safety.

Take Home Point: The TFP contract process will address the ways psychiatric hospitalization can interfere with the treatment and ways psychiatric hospitalization can preserve the treatment.

5.3   The TFP Contract Explores in Advance Specific Contingencies Related to Psychiatric Hospitalization

> - *The TFP contracting phase will include explicit discussion of the possibility of psychiatric hospitalization.*
> - *The TFP contract will anticipate treatment-interfering behaviors that may require inpatient hospitalization.*
> - *The TFP contract clarifies in advance that the individual therapist will not interfere with emergency room or inpatient clinicians' decision-making.*
> - *The TFP contract will anticipate the possibility that inpatient hospitalization* itself *may be a treatment-interfering behavior.*

The TFP contract is understood as acting as a "third party" of sorts for the clinician offering treatment to the patient with serious personality disorder pathology. The contract offers the clinician a "port in the storm" during the period of affective intensity – a solid set of reference points during periods that can often threaten the clinician's ability to think clearly and act helpfully.

The inpatient psychiatric hospitalization in today's climate is axiomatically associated with heightened affective intensity for patients with PD symptoms, given the relatively high barriers to hospitalization now routine in this country. To this end, the TFP contract prepares the patient, family, and therapist in advance for the thorny process of hospitalization. In the contracting phase, the therapist will go to lengths to explore the patient's prior treatment history, including the patient's prior hospitalizations. Just as the therapist is highly motivated to learn about the patient's prior individual treatment experiences, with the goal of elucidating the likely object relations dyads activated in those relationships, so too will the history of prior hospitalizations shed light on the patient's experience of self and others, very likely to repeat in the TFP treatment.

In the TFP contracting phase, the therapist will not accept at face value a patient's reassurance that past behaviors that may have interfered with useful psychotherapy have completely resolved. The TFP therapist will engage the patient in an extensive discussion of "What if?" a particular symptom or behavior might recur. To this point, the therapist will want to flesh out in advance the possibility that a certain symptom – self-injurious or suicidal acts, substance use, eating disorder symptoms, etc. – not necessarily in evidence in the evaluation period, could return and possibly require inpatient level of care to insure the patient's safety temporarily.

The TFP therapist will have uppermost in mind after beginning treatment the potential that certain of the patient's behaviors could undermine the treatment and therefore the patient's stated goals. This is not because patients enjoy undermining treatment. It is rather that a psychotherapy that explores a patient's inner world inevitably leads to thoughts and feels that are disturbing – the very thoughts and feelings that the patient's primitive defenses attempt to avoid. Therefore, the behaviors that might undermine the treatment can be best thought of as resistances to exploration of the mind. The goal will always be to have the patient return to treatment, if it is possible for both the patient and therapist to feel safe doing so, and to have an opportunity to explore the contributions to the emergence of treatment-threatening behavior, particularly in the context of the transference.

The TFP therapist in the contracting phase describes a well-defined and limited role should the patient present for evaluation to the emergency department or be admitted to the inpatient psychiatric unit. This well-defined role of the therapist may feel depriving to many patients who have experienced prior therapists' active involvement as evidence of "caring" and professionalism. This part of the TFP contract implicitly confronts a patient's experience of the therapist as omniscient or omnipresent and the patient's experience of self as incapable of effective action. The patient is made aware in advance that the emergency room clinicians will decide whether to hold, admit, or discharge the patient, as only they are in a position to provide the patient with a thorough assessment at that point in time. The TFP therapist will, in a similar vein, defer to the inpatient team regarding most key decisions in the patient's treatment. The TFP therapist may see a hospitalized patient on the unit if possible, but the TFP therapist, mindful of the risk of "secondary gain" or sense of gratification from extra attention obtained through a maladaptive mechanism like hospitalization, will limit those visits and not attempt to conduct "intensive therapy" while the patient is on the unit. Clear, unambivalent discussion of this approach with patients and families *during the contracting phase* will address in advance the risk of an outsized reaction on the part of the patient and/or family reflecting an experience of the therapist as negligent or uncaring.

In general, the TFP therapist regards a psychiatric hospitalization as neither inherently positive nor negative. In this role, the TFP therapist confronts commonly observed emerging dyads in consideration of hospitalization: the patient idealizing the hospitalization as limitlessly nurturing and benign or, alternatively, the patient regarding the hospital with paranoia, expecting sadism, incompetence, or a combination of the two. The TFP therapist will feel confident endorsing a hospitalization for certain specific purposes. Those purposes can include revisiting the patient's diagnosis with the input of the inpatient team. Another reasonable goal would be to make adjustments in the patient's medication regimen, if those adjustments can only safely be accomplished in such a setting. The therapist will endorse a hospitalization if a patient's symptoms escalate to the point that useful therapy is not possible – as with the patient with an eating disorder, whose weight loss causes medical instability or a diminished capacity for focus, or the substance-using patient, whose attendance in treatment and mental clarity are compromised. For clinicians reluctant to share with patients a personality disorder diagnosis they have made with confidence, but fear conveying, the inpatient hospital setting may confer the security and support the clinician needs to do so. The inpatient hospitalization may be an ideal setting for family psychoeducation, including a review of the diagnosis and frank discussion of prognosis.

The TFP therapist is also aware that psychiatric hospitalization itself can be a treatment-interfering behavior. A patient's hospitalization early in TFP treatment may reflect the patient's "testing" of the therapist to see if he or she will follow through with the contract as has been stated. A hospitalization can serve as a "protest" about the TFP contract's expectation for meaningful work or studies. The patient may also unconsciously seek hospitalization to humiliate the therapist in the community, to show that the therapist has not been helpful or even has done harm, as an expression of aggression or sadism in the transference.

Ms. A. Expects Her Psychiatrist to Intervene on Her Behalf When She Is Evaluated in the Emergency Room for Possible Psychiatric Hospitalization

Clinical vignette: When Ms. A. was an undergraduate, she was twice evaluated in the emergency room near the campus following overdoses of her prescription medications after arguments with her boyfriend. Both times, representatives of the college's student health center came to the emergency room to be with Ms. A. and actively advocated for her release from the hospital, despite the concerns of the attending psychiatrist on call. Ms. A. found the support of the counseling service staff to be highly gratifying and felt they "saved" her from the callous, uncaring hospital staff.

After graduation Ms. A. begins treatment with Dr. Y. who explains that he believes the overdoses and Ms. A.'s continued unstable mood reflect a personality disorder diagnosis and not the "atypical bipolar" diagnosis she

(continued)

(continued)

had been given in the past. Dr. Y. explains to Ms. A. that should she become suicidal going forward, he would not intervene with either emergency department or inpatient psychiatry clinicians' decision-making. Ms. A. and her mother, who joins her for a meeting with Dr. Y. early in the treatment, express surprise at this approach but accept Dr. Y.'s policy.

Six months later Ms. A. finds out her new boyfriend may be cheating on her. She leaves a panicked message for Dr. Y. in the middle of the night before taking five Ambien tablets and calling 911. The next morning Dr. Y. is contacted by the emergency department and by Ms. A.'s mother. Ms. A.'s mother reports that her daughter is frantic to leave the hospital emergency department as soon as possible so as not to miss work at her new job. Ms. A. wants Dr. Y. to instruct the emergency department staff to let her go immediately. Dr. Y. reminds Ms. A.'s mother about his policy and goes over it again a few hours later with Ms. A. herself when she calls from the hospital.

When Ms. A. comes for her next appointment, she is unusually sullen and quiet. Dr. Y. asks Ms. A. if this may be a reaction to his response to calls from the emergency department, and Ms. A. acknowledges it is. What follows is a an extended discussion of Ms. A.'s concerns that Dr. Y. may not care for her as she had hoped he might, as revealed by his unwillingness to advocate for her. Dr. Y. reiterates that he feels having Ms. A.'s care managed during off hours by those available at the emergency department does in fact reflect concern, but not the kind of rescue Ms. A. might wish. Ms. A. grudgingly accepts that this may be the case.

Take Home Point: The TFP therapist will remain aware of the risk that the patient's desire to have the therapist intervene during emergencies can reflect the "secondary gain" of eliciting attention or care.

5.4 TFP Principles Can Guide Outpatient Clinicians in Decision-Making About Psychiatric Hospitalization

- *The clinician's decision-making process about hospitalization will often be more complicated with PD patients than it is with patients from other diagnostic groups.*
- *TFP principles can help clinicians making decisions about hospitalization for the PD patient with suicidality, a familiar and unnerving challenge.*
- *TFP principles can aid clinicians making decisions about hospitalizing PD patients, even when those clinicians do not have a long-standing or clearly defined relationship with the patient.*

The therapist's quandary about the utility of a psychiatric hospitalization for the patient with PD symptomatology is particularly fraught and with good reason. Because of the powerful transference and countertransference currents so often seen in treatment with this population, the decision-making about hospitalization can be complicated for and even disturbing to the therapist. Clinicians understandably find decision-making about hospitalization in the context of a patient's suicidality a particularly challenging situation.

Clinicians can make decisions about hospitalization when evaluating patients with certain diagnoses based purely on widely accepted treatment algorithms. One example is that of an emergency room psychiatrist evaluating a patient she does not know who presents with major depression with emerging mood-congruent psychotic thinking. The psychiatrist requires the patient be hospitalized and makes this decision without ambivalence. When this same clinician evaluates a patient with borderline personality traits presenting to the emergency room with more ambiguous symptoms (self-injurious but denying suicidality, refusing a voluntary admission but describing impairment in self-care), her countertransference may be marked by confusion and self-doubt, in contrast to the sense of certainty and competence she felt evaluating the depressed patient. TFP principles may be useful in the emergency room in a case like this, even when the clinician does not have an enduring relationship with the patient.

The use of TFP principles may confer for outpatient therapists a set of "blueprints" for this process. As noted, there are a number of very good reasons for the therapist to strongly recommend or even require a psychiatric hospitalization for a patient. In TFP, the goal is twofold: one, to address any co-occurring conditions or behavior that could undermine the treatment and two, to insure that both the patient and therapist are able to feel safe and secure in the treatment in a way that supports useful work toward the patient's goals.

The TFP therapist will be asking: What is the meaning of hospitalization in the transference? What dyads are activated leading to behaviors or symptoms requiring hospitalization, and/or what dyads are activated by the process of hospitalization? What is the therapist's countertransference and how might this influence decision-making?

Much of the literature on hospitalization of patients with BPD focuses on the risk of unnecessary hospitalizations [10]. In the typical case, the clinician is moved to hospitalize the patient in the context of an inadequately examined countertransference reaction, often related to a patient's suicidality. For example, the therapist who allows a sadistic patient to taunt her with subtle threats of suicide becomes exhausted and abruptly calls for emergency services, even though she does not believe the patient will act on the threats or that hospitalization will be of use to the patient. Another scenario is the therapist who fears introduction of explicit negativity in the transference and arranges hospitalization as a way to placate a distressed patient and assist the patient in avoiding difficult realities in her life. The TFP approach, with its persistent focus on countertransference reactions, can help the therapist negotiate these tricky situations and avoid counterproductive hospitalizations.

In some of these cases, TFP principles can assist clinicians who may be *reluctant* to hospitalize a patient. As noted, patients may often become paranoid about a possible hospitalization and ascribe to the therapist sadistic impulses in encouraging one. Take the example of a patient who has been evasive about his abuse of benzodiazepines and developed a level of tolerance that would make an outpatient taper impossible. The therapist using TFP principles would invoke the contract to push for a hospitalization that would safely address this issue and put into place an appropriate outpatient treatment plan that would, in time, allow the patient to continue in individual psychotherapy without the interference of an active substance use disorder. The TFP therapist, who remains focused on the overarching goal of aiding the patient in making character-altering changes through the use of the psychotherapy, will be in a better position to tolerate objections or even accusations when recommending hospitalization as described. Remaining mindful of longer-term goals can anchor the therapist negotiating the doubt and confusion that can accompany the process of decision-making in relation to hospitalization of the PD patient.

The clinician who has some responsibility for making decisions about hospitalizing a patient with personality disorder symptoms, but not necessarily a clearly defined or enduring relationship with this patient, can also use TFP thinking as part of the calculus about the decision. This is a familiar scenario in the emergency department. This, of course, does not pertain to those situations where the decision-making is clear – as in the case of a patient with the neurovegetative signs and symptoms of depression in combination with suicidal ideation, but as noted, with PD patients, this is often not the case. The clinician in the ER (or IOP or partial program or on consultation-liaison service) asks the same questions: What is the diagnosis? How am I feeling and what does that mean? What is going on in the patient's key relationships right now, including with a primary therapist and with me? What can I do or say to address the active relationships and could it change the decision-making process about hospitalization?

Dr. C. Evaluates a Suicidal Outpatient and Makes a Decision About Hospitalization

Clinical vignette: Dr. C. works at an inner-city municipal hospital emergency department providing psychiatric evaluation services for a large partial hospital program (PHP) serving patients with chronic and disabling conditions. The PHP includes volunteer work opportunities for patients on disability who want support in moving toward paid employment.

PHP staff bring in Ms. N., a middle-aged woman well known to them for many months, because of their concern about her escalating suicidality. Ms. N. had been hospitalized numerous times in her mid-20s, but now at age 40, she was fully engaged at the PHP, working 30 hours weekly at the volunteer program and planning to begin applying for jobs as a receptionist with a goal of returning to full employment.

Dr. C. reviews Ms. N.'s extensive record that gives her primary diagnosis as social anxiety disorder. Dr. C. is struck by Ms. N.'s current crisis, increased suicidality because of perceived rejection by a staff member at the PHP, and her level of chronic disability, which Dr. C. does not feel is fully accounted for by a social anxiety disorder diagnosis. In her evaluation of Ms. N., Dr. C. notes Ms. N.'s long-standing history of spotty employment and unstable relationships, suggestive of significant identity diffusion, with frequent ruptures in treatment, associated with the kind of perceived rejection that has led to the current crisis, reflecting compromised coping mechanisms. During their initial interview, Dr. C. is aware of her own lack of sympathy for and irritation with Ms. N., despite Ms. N.'s superficial tearfulness and despair – a lack of sympathy likely related to the patient's otherwise general calm and subtle air of satisfaction.

Dr. C. attempts to clarify the events leading to Ms. N.'s recent suicidality, learning that Ms. N. became angry with

(continued)

(continued)

her therapist at the PHP when the therapist announced she would be going on maternity leave later that year. Dr. C. considers a dominant dyad of abandoned, powerless patient and uncaring therapist, alternating with one of powerful patient whose threats of suicide control her flailing therapist.

Dr. C. approaches Ms. N. and explains her own thinking about hospitalization: "You could come into the hospital, but I would be concerned about the disruption to your volunteer position, and the risk of setting back your job search. I am aware that you only recently became suicidal after hearing about your therapist's upcoming leave. I would guess that leaves you feeling hurt and without resources. I am also aware that your threats of suicide had a big impact on your therapist and the staff at your program, that you 'turned the tables' and became the one calling the shots."

Ms. N.'s presentation changing from a mix of despairing and satisfied to curious and concerned responds: "I don't want to lose my volunteer job and I want to start going on interviews, but losing my therapist for 3 months will be devastating." Dr. N. replies, "Coming into the hospital may temporarily help you feel like you're back in control, but it has risks. Feeling suicidal may be your way of managing the loss, but the consequences of hospitalization are real and concerning." Ms. N. is able to negotiate a release from the emergency department back to her treatment team at the PHP. Dr. C. documents her diagnostic impression (including personality disorder traits), her thinking about the risks and benefits of hospitalization, and her discussion with the PHP staff about Ms. N.'s interpersonally-mediated mood reactivity and how this may differ from a social anxiety disorder diagnosis.

Take Home Point: The outpatient clinician charged with making a decision about hospitalizing a suicidal patient with personality disorder pathology can use TFP interventions including "naming the actors" to manage the process.

5.5   TFP Principles Can Help Minimize the Risks of Psychiatric Hospitalization

- *The hospitalization of patients with severe PD symptoms is associated with significant risks.*
- *Splitting between outpatient and inpatient clinicians and among inpatient clinicians is a common, expectable problem.*
- *The inpatient team will likely be subject to intense pressures and alternating idealization or devaluation that can lead to excessive "action."*
- *TFP's focus on diagnosis, predominant defenses employed, and dyads activated can help clinicians limit those risks associated with hospitalization.*

The hospitalization of patients with PD diagnoses can be associated with significant risks, well described in the literature, and those risks can have outcomes, in many cases, at cross-purposes with TFP's essential goals. To repeat, the TFP therapist will not reflexively support or contest a hospitalization but will be vigilant about the associated risks, among them: (1) the patient's regression in the hospital setting, (2) derailment of the patient's life outside the hospital and loss of important social supports at work or school, (3) "contagion" in the hospital setting including self-injury and eating disorder symptoms, and (4) counterproductive interventions by hospital staff including questionable polypharmacy or electroconvulsive therapy (ECT).

The TFP therapist's contract is designed to minimize the risks described. TFP's prioritization of patient autonomy can be undermined by a regressing hospitalization associated with a patient's loss of the social structure of work or school. The TFP therapist would not "reward" the hospitalized patient with excessive attention, but rather will communicate that continued work in treatment after hospitalization, in the office setting consistent with the contract's defined treatment frame, would be optimal. A patient can be influenced during a hospitalization to experiment with maladaptive mechanisms for self-regulation, like novel forms or self-injury or eating disorders. These new symptoms then become additionally concerning treatment-interfering behaviors, sometimes adding to the maladaptive behaviors that led to the hospitalization in the first place. Patients with PD diagnoses with or without co-occurring mood or anxiety disorders will sometimes leave the hospital with a particularly complicated medication regimen; at times, the medication side effects of this regimen (e.g., excessive sedation, insomnia, agitation) can add to a patient's limitations in functioning, despite the best intentions of the inpatient prescribers.

The inpatient psychiatry team in these times juggles a number of demands: (1) administrators want to keep lengths of stay relatively brief, (2) payers expect treatments with a rapid response, and (3) patients, families, and outside treaters often wish for a treatment milieu or effective brief psychotherapeutic interventions unavailable on today's mostly "medical model" units. The inpatient team will often feel compelled to act in these circumstances, sometimes with recommendations for complex polypharmacy or even ECT in some cases.

During a hospitalization, the patient's primitive defenses can engender splitting among involved treaters, be it between outpatient and inpatient clinicians or on the hospital unit among members of the inpatient treatment team. This frequently lamented phenomenon nonetheless seems to repeat itself with clockwise regularity [11]. It is important to remember that a patient with a split psychological organization is not *either* a misunderstood victim or an angry bully, but is alternately *both*. The TFP therapist's understanding of this pattern of splitting identifies the conflicts between outpatient and inpatient treaters, or among staff on the inpatient unit, as an externalization of the patient's internal conflict. Sometimes the hospitalized patient will appear counterintuitively serene, while members of the treatment team or outpatient and inpatient clinicians skirmish among themselves. The risk if this splitting process continues unchecked, of course, is that the patient would not grapple with critical internal conflicts that likely contributed to the need for hospitalization in the first place.

The TFP model may assist clinicians in avoiding the risks described, using the process of (1) diagnostic clarification, including consideration of personality disorder pathology, (2) appreciation of specific defenses employed as part of a diagnostic assessment, and (3) exploration of predictably activated dyads and their reverses, and appreciation of the links between these dyads, and the factors contributing to hospitalization.

It may seem obvious but the outpatient clinician's clear communication with the inpatient staff about a patient's diagnoses is critical and influential. The inpatient staff will likely be reluctant to prioritize a personality disorder diagnosis, given their limited time with the patient and external pressures to justify the higher inpatient level of care. *The inpatient staff may need a direct, detailed communication about a PD diagnosis at the outset of a hospitalization, with a specific, clearly articulated description of the risks for a particular patient, informed by diagnostic thinking.* The outpatient therapist's understanding of a patient's specific pattern of defenses utilized should underscore those risks often observed, as with a patient's pattern of: (1) splitting (through alternating idealization and devaluation), (2) omnipotent control, (3) projection or projective identification, or (4) denial, often in combination. Yet even with this communication of information, an approach to patient treatment that does not fit a narrow "medical model" may be alien to inpatient teams.

In fact, in the treatment of patients with PD diagnoses, inpatient and outpatient treaters alike are compelled to consider the *entire* continuum of symptom expression from the most obviously biologic to the most obviously psychodynamic manifestation of the disorder, with all of the possible permutations in between. The defining goal of any hospitalization is the identification of an effective multimodal treatment, as is strongly supported by research [12]. Given contemporary understanding of personality disorder pathology, a distinction made by any clinician between a "biologic" and "psychodynamic" approach is at once specious and anachronistic. In one typical, concerning pattern, a "split" emerges between inpatient and outpatient treaters, often cast as a reflection of dueling "biologic" and "psychodynamic" orientations. (Inpatient treaters are often, although not always, seen as identifying with the "biologic" orientation, in part because of the pressures they are under to institute treatments rapidly because of present-day time constraints.) Clinicians finding themselves at odds either within a particular team or as part of "competing" teams in the treatment of a PD patient will benefit from considering to what extent differences of opinion reflect aspects of the psychological make-up of the patient in question rather than truly consequential differing theoretical orientations.

How would the outpatient and inpatient treaters' understanding of "primitive" defensive operations contribute to limitation of adverse effects from a hospitalization? Splitting may be observed as a patient's alternating idealization and devaluation of others, including treaters. How would this impact a hospitalization? One common story is the patient who actively resists the therapist's recommendation for hospitalization, often suspicious or frankly paranoid about the suggestion, fearing a one-dimensionally "bad" inpatient staff. This patient may, after admission, exhibit a profound shift, now experiencing the staff as caring and helpful in an idealized way and then making discharge from the hospital problematic. This vignette captures the splitting defense (alternating devaluation and idealization) and the oscillation of dyads (powerful treater "mistreating" vulnerable patient to empowered patient controlling hapless clinicians). The outpatient therapist and inpatient team, both appreciative of the patient's defensive operations and associated experiences of self and others, would be more likely to work together in an effective and coordinated fashion.

Outpatient and inpatient treaters are understandably confused when a patient admitted to the hospital restricts the flow of information between them. Common sense would suggest that a patient requiring an inpatient level of care would want to have all those involved in her care – family, outpatient treaters, and inpatient team – communicating freely; clinicians working with patients with severe PD pathology, however, know well that this is not always the case. The inpatient treatment team aware in advance of the PD patient's pattern of using defenses such as omnipotent control (an unconscious motivation to insure safety by controlling others) might address such controlling behavior proactively. How might this work? Imagine the inpatient nurse or psychiatrist taking the patient's history on admission. How would the clinician react if the patient became angry or even paranoid at the request for contact with the outpatient team? In this situation, the inpatient staff can follow the tactic the TFP therapist in the outpatient setting may routinely take when a disruptive expression of omnipotent control is evident. The therapist would identify the dyad (vulnerable patient, intrusive or even threatening treater) and its reverse (empowered patient, vulnerable clinician left "in the dark") and then describe this pattern to the patient. The inpatient treater might do the same. First identify the dyad in play and its reverse, and then articulate this observation to the patient, as in this case: "You seem fearful that if I reach out to your treatment team and your family I might use this information against you. It's as if you feel powerless and with this information I might be empowered to hurt you. But I'm aware at the same time you're in control, deciding who I speak to or don't speak to, leaving me not fully informed and more tentative than I might be." This approach would address a pattern of resistance to exploration, discussed above as a major motivator of acting out and defensive behavior.

The defenses of projection and projective identification have some common elements but some important differences. The patient using the defense of projection cannot tolerate awareness of two sides of a conflict and may, when interacting with a clinician, attribute unacceptable attitudes not fully in the patient's awareness *to* the clinician. One example is that a patient is admitted to the hospital in crisis, but superficially defiant, after it is revealed she is having an affair, threatening her marriage. On intake, as the social worker is professionally gathering history, the patient bursts out: "You think I'm a bad mother because of this affair I'm describing!" The social worker monitors her countertransference and because she does not have a particularly judgmental attitude toward the patient begins to speculate that the patient's outburst reflects some intolerable feeling about herself. Projection is understood as a repression-based defense, used by a variety of patients across the spectrum of functioning, in contrast to projective identification, largely considered a splitting-based defense. How might projective identification work in the inpatient setting and why is it important to appreciate? Here is a typical sequence of events: (1) The patient has a disavowed or uncomfortable-making part of himself, (2) the patient induces this feeling in his therapist, and (3) the patient identifies this feeling in the therapist and reacts, sometimes strongly, often by needing to control the therapist. The therapist who actively monitors his/her countertransference may identify an uncharacteristic thought or feeling in response to a patient in this context, reflecting this process outlined. Take the example of a patient with borderline and narcissistic traits, persistently symptomatic and prone to blaming prescribers for "not getting the medications right." This patient has a pattern of "externalizing" his internal conflicts, in this case making his difficulties in functioning about others' (his prescribers') failures. How might this patient, when hospitalized, employ projective identification and how might this unfold? The disavowed or uncomfortable-making affect for this patient may be covert sadism; the patient may induce this in his treaters in a way that sometimes enters the treater's awareness (as in: "Why do I feel so hateful toward this patient? Why don't I care if the medications I prescribe cause unpleasant side effects? Why do I feel unmotivated to make recommendations for medication changes?"). The hypothesis about projective identification would account for (1) the therapist's uncharacteristic countertransference reaction and (2) the patient's response to the clinician's experience of sadism as in: "Why are you suggesting this intervention (medication, ECT) that will destroy me?" or "Why are you denying me medication that will make me feel better?" This might explain the common counterintuitive process of the PD patient's reflexive rejection of possibly helpful changes in medication *or* inexplicable total acquiescence to an unwieldy medication regimen of multiple agents with multiple side effects.

In the past, a patient with severe PD symptomatology might exhibit the defensive operation of denial by engaging in behaviors guaranteeing a long-term psychiatric hospitalization, free from responsibilities of everyday life, keeping out of his or her awareness the realities of months of missed school or work, financial pressures associated with the hospitalization, or the impact of the hospitalization on spouse, children, or extended family. This may no longer be possible as it once was, but patients today can still use hospitalization in this way, to temporarily keep split apart two emotionally distinct areas of awareness. An example is a patient with BPD who comes into the hospital after an overdose. The patient seems generally unruffled by this episode, appearing cheerful and sociable on the unit. At the same time, the patient's absence from work is jeopardizing her family's financial situation, causing marked distress for her husband and children.

The Inpatient Treatment Team Grapples with the Difficulties Caused by the Patient Whose Behavior Divides the Staff

Clinical vignette: Dr. E., a psychiatrist, and Mr. J., a social worker, are newly assigned staff at an "affective disorders" inpatient unit. Dr. E. and Mr. J. expect the population of this unit to have clinical presentations reflecting primary mood and anxiety disorder diagnoses, but quickly they find the diagnoses of the patients to be more

(continued)

(continued)

variable and complicated than they had anticipated. Initially they see their patients on the unit individually, but soon they realize they are often finding themselves with a different understanding of certain patients, leading to confusion and some tension between them.

The admission of Ms. O. brings this situation to a head. Ms. O., a single woman in her late 20s, had been hospitalized on this unit twice during the past year. During those hospitalizations, the unit's nursing staff found Ms. O. to be unpleasant and often untrustworthy, while the medical staff found her to be sympathetic. These divergent impressions led to some heated discussions in rounds, particularly when Ms. O. requested passes as part of her discharge planning, felt by the nursing staff to be concerning and premature, but readily endorsed by the medical staff, who found Ms. O. to be cooperative and engaged.

Dr. E. and Mr. J. review Ms. O.'s record at the time of her readmission, which suggests that her two admissions in the previous year represented exacerbations of long-standing depression and social anxiety disorder. Those admissions had been precipitated by Ms. O.'s threats of suicide, when she had become despondent after she was threatened with firing from her job as a secretary.

At the time of this latest admission, Ms. O. had only recently started treatment with a new outpatient team, a social worker therapist and a nurse practitioner prescriber. Her therapist directly contacts Dr. E. and Mr. J. at the time of Ms. O.s' hospitalization and goes to some lengths to describe her diagnostic impression: a primary personality disorder with borderline and "thin-skinned" narcissistic traits, a secondary depressive disorder, not

(continued)

(continued)

likely to be improved significantly with medications, and sensitivity to perceived rejection, more likely attributable to the narcissistic traits identified than a distinct anxiety disorder. Ms. O.'s therapist also outlines her understanding of Ms. O.'s problematic coping strategies including a pattern, not in her awareness, of pitting important people in her life against each other, controlling others through her behaviors, and ascribing to others intolerable aspects of herself, particularly aspects of her disavowed aggression.

In the first 24 hours of Ms. O.'s hospitalization, she is deferential to Dr. E. but dismissive of Mr. J. She gives Mr. J. "orders" about what kind of discharge plans she will require, listing a number of requests that would take him many hours of investigation to deliver. Dr. E. and Mr. J. meet and compare their differing experiences with Ms. O. and explore how they imagine Ms. O.'s diagnostic profile, as described by her new therapist, might contribute to the behaviors (friction between nurses and doctors, controlling demands about discharge planning) already observed.

Dr. E. and Mr. J. decide to hold their daily meetings with Ms. O. together. Quickly this alters the discrepant reactions to the patient they previously had experienced. They work in tandem with Ms. O.'s outpatient treaters to avoid an extended stay in the hospital that might reinforce Ms. O.'s problematic and self-defeating way of coping with the perceived humiliation at her job.

Take Home Point: Inpatient clinicians open to making a personality disorder diagnosis can adjust treatment interventions that will preserve staff unity and help the staff avoid introduction of iatrogenic complications.

5.6   TFP Principles Can Maximize the Benefits of Psychiatric Hospitalization

> - *TFP principles support hospitalization in certain situations, often with the aim of addressing treatment-threatening behavior.*
> - *Hospitalization goals can include: clarifying diagnosis, evaluating factors contributing to a serious suicide attempt, reviewing a medication regimen, and addressing co-occurring conditions or adding adjunctive treatments.*
> - *The TFP therapist may use the hospitalization to clarify the patient's commitment to the treatment or consider alternatives.*
> - *Inpatient staff can use TFP principles adapted for their short-term, high-acuity setting when working with PD patients.*

The TFP therapist will endorse a psychiatric hospitalization when the goals of the hospitalization line up with those of the treatment. As already noted, the goals of hospitalization are often related to addressing any emerging situation or behavior that might impair the ability of the patient and therapist to continue in treatment safely and productively. Sometimes a hospitalization will lead to a suspension of the treatment. This could occur when a patient with a restrictive eating disorder develops medical instability, as determined by an internist, and requires a period of specialized treatment before returning to TFP. Another situation might be the patient with a chronic dysphoria of a personality disorder who develops clear neurovegetative symptoms and mood-congruent delusional preoccupations. This presentation would require a hospitalization and focused treatment before revisiting the possibility of restarting this particular psychotherapy.

There are other times when the TFP therapist might strongly recommend a psychiatric hospitalization. This might occur when the therapist begins to question a patient's diagnosis and feels an inpatient hospitalization, with access to specialized testing and the built-in consultation/second opinion input of the inpatient staff, would be beneficial. One possibility might be the patient thought to have a primary personality disorder whose micro-psychotic episodes become more sustained and concerning. In this case, an inpatient hospitalization to revisit diagnosis, assess for organic causes for these changes, and possibly initiate antipsychotic medication might be indicated.

A serious life-threatening suicide attempt would be another indication for a psychiatric hospitalization. All clinicians treating patients with severe personality disorders develop a line of inquiry, with the goal of clarifying aspects of suicidal behavior, which assesses details about means, intent, timing, and lethality, among other subjects. The TFP therapist would support a hospitalization after a serious suicide attempt with a goal of understanding the details of the event (in particular in the context of developments in the transference), examining the action in terms of the patient's diagnostic presentation (especially evidence of biological vs. characterological depression), and considering changes in the patient's level of care and treatment plan. One profile in this category would be the patient thought to have a personality disorder diagnosis whose suicide attempt is closely linked with an active, but unacknowledged, substance use disorder. The opportunity to use time in the hospital to review with a patient findings of a toxicology screen and to investigate a previously covert alcohol, recreational drug, or prescription drug misuse pattern could be productive and even life-saving.

Polypharmacy is a hallmark of treatment for BPD, and patients with other PD diagnoses too can be prescribed multiple medications, often with limited effectiveness and substantial risk [13, 14]. All medications prescribed for PD symptoms are done so "off label," and in recent years the range of medication types used with PD patients has expanded [15].

A psychiatric hospitalization to review a patient's medication regimen may be indicated if the medication regimen in question cannot be safely adjusted in outpatient treatment. One such story involves a patient presenting for psychotherapy because of the deterioration of her marriage; the patient herself is a physician and she is taking medication samples (antidepressants, atypical antipsychotics), while prescribed multiple sedative-hypnotics for sleep by a primary care physician whom she sees irregularly. In this case the complexity of the patient's regimen and the amount and variety of sedative-hypnotic medications she is taking make a hospitalization, as part of preparation for an extended individual psychotherapy, imperative.

The TFP therapist is open to the addition of adjunctive treatments when those treatments are understood as likely helpful for the patient in attaining personal and psychotherapy goals. The TFP therapist can use a hospitalization to assess fully a patient's co-occurring conditions and initiate appropriate adjunctive interventions. These adjunctive interventions can include substance use support groups, marital or family counseling, or targeted cognitive-behavioral treatment focusing on a specific symptom.

The inpatient hospitalization can sometimes be used to assess the patient's motivation for TFP treatment. There may be circumstances when a patient in crisis makes a decision to identify another treatment, when it becomes clear that, for either logistical reasons (cost or scheduling) or a change in the patient's motivation, the TFP format is no longer possible. The inpatient setting may be the place to confirm that a patient does not have the interest in psychological exploration expected in TFP. When the patient in TFP is in the hospital and it is determined that TFP may not be the treatment of choice for whatever reason, the focus of the inpatient stay may then shift to identifying another better suited treatment modality.

The inpatient psychiatrist familiar with central TFP concepts can use elements of TFP even when the patients in question are not, nor will be, patients in extended, exploratory psychotherapies. The inpatient clinician can use these core TFP concepts when assessing and treating inpatients including:

1. A systematic diagnostic process that includes exploration of personality traits/structure and levels of functioning
2. Comfort with engaging patients and families in discussion of personality disorder symptoms in their various manifestations
3. Appreciation of defenses, including the more primitive splitting-based operations
4. The concept of the patient taking responsibility for certain behaviors and certain aspects of his/her treatment
5. Identification of key dyads and their inverses

An openness to the three channels of communication, with a particular sensitivity to countertransference reactions, including splits within the team, can aid inpatient clinicians when taking this approach.

In comparison to clinicians on consultation-liaison services or in emergency departments, inpatient treaters may have more time to perform a systematic diagnostic interview with patients that could include an extended exploration of defenses and levels of functioning. The inpatient treater can sometimes meet with a patient successively over days in the assessment process, while obtaining parallel information from outpatient treaters and family members. The clinician with the benefit of an extended, thorough evaluation may be more likely to entertain a personality disorder diagnosis, particularly when the clinician is prompted by the structural interview format. Clinicians in general may feel more comfortable introducing the topic of a personality disorder diagnosis when patients are in secure, inpatient settings. The additional supervision of the inpatient service may allow clinicians to discuss diagnostic issues they had previously avoided out of concern about the patient's risk for suicide or intense anger in response. The more likely involvement of family during a patient's inpatient stay can present to both outpatient and inpatient clinicians an opportunity to explore diagnosis, prognosis, and additional psychoeducation opportunities available for families of patients with personality disorders.

The highly stimulating inpatient setting will likely quickly bring to the surface a patient's use of more maladaptive defenses. The inpatient staff, aware of this possibility and armed with a shorthand for these patterns, can avoid certain predictable and unproductive interventions. The staff will be attuned to patterns of splitting (alternating idealization and devaluation, causing rifts among staff members), projective identification (leading staff to experience unsettling feelings such as guilt or anger not tolerated by the patient), omnipotent control (patients' actions controlling staff, thereby limiting their effectiveness), and denial (keeping difficult realities at bay, making regression in the hospital more comfortable). Inpatient staff can manage these challenging situations by identifying the activated dyads and putting the patient's experience into words. This process of diagnostic questioning, identification of defenses, and explication of dyads gives inpatient clinicians a grounding way to approach patients.

Ms. F. Is Readmitted and Dr. R. Wants to Avoid the Derailment and Regression that Were Part of Her Prior Hospitalization

Clinical vignette: Dr. R. is a psychologist working in a state hospital general psychiatry inpatient unit. The hospital's population includes the chronically mentally ill, as well as patients admitted with episodic illness, some of whom have prominent personality disorder symptoms.

Ms. F., a single woman in her late 20s, is readmitted to Dr. R.'s service following a suicide attempt by overdose. Ms. F. had been under Dr. R.'s care during an extended hospitalization the previous year, one Dr. R. considered to be counterproductive. During that hospitalization

(continued)

(continued)

Ms. F. lost her job as a teacher, requiring her to borrow money from her parents after a number of years of financial independence. The unit's psychiatry resident found Ms. F. to be highly sympathetic and earnest, while the nursing staff found her to be dismissive and rude, resulting in some friction during rounds. The hospitalization lasted almost 6 weeks, much longer than Dr. R. had felt necessary, as Ms. F. suggested and then refused a range of outpatient treatment opportunities, including specific programs and providers. In addition, Ms. F.'s persistent complaints of insomnia led the unit's psychiatrist to use a sedating atypical antipsychotic medication for both sleep disturbance and as an adjunct to her depression regimen, causing her to gain 50 pounds in the 1-year period between hospitalizations. At the time of Ms. F.'s initial admission, the team had entertained a personality disorder diagnosis (with borderline and dependent traits), but the unit director had felt strongly that no personality disorder could be made reliably while Ms. O. reported continued depression symptoms.

Dr. R.'s assessment of Ms. F. at the time of her readmission was notable for an absence of neurovegetative symptoms in the weeks prior to her suicide attempt and a clear association between her overdose and an argument between Ms. F. and her parents. Dr. R. feels strongly that Ms. F.'s history and current presentation reflect a primary personality disorder diagnosis and with this in mind presents in rounds his diagnostic impression and goals for the hospitalization.

In rounds, Dr. R. outlines the following goals, informed by Ms. F.'s personality disorder diagnosis: clarification of the severity of her suicide attempt; discussion with Ms. F. and her outpatient treaters of the contribution of personality disorder symptoms to her current picture; involvement of Ms. F.'s parents in this discussion, given her

(continued)

*dependence on their emotional and financial support;
and a reexamination of her medication regimen, with a
plan to taper those agents with limited efficacy and/or
troubling side effects. Dr. R. also includes a prediction
that Ms. F.'s behavior may cause dissension among the
staff; he encourages the staff to adopt a coordinated
approach to Ms. F.'s care to limit this distraction.*

*Dr. R. and the unit staff are able to use Ms. F.'s time on
the inpatient service productively. A discussion of personality disorder symptoms and associated defenses res-
onates with the staff, putting into words aspects of the
patient's behavior and their reactions that had been present, but not well defined. Working in coordination allows
the team to address the issues of diagnosis, family psychoeducation, and reduction in medications with less
conflict than they had anticipated. They accomplish their
goals and discharge Ms. F. in a timely manner.*

*Take Home Point: Clarity of diagnostic thinking and
staff coordination are essential elements in maximizing
the benefit of an inpatient hospitalization for the patient
with severe personality disorder pathology.*

References

1. Nelson KJ. Managing borderline personality disorder on general psychiatry units. Psychdyn Psychiatry. 2013;41(4):563–74.
2. Paris J. Treatment of borderline personality disorder: a guide to evidence-based practice. New York: NY Guilford Press; 2008.
3. Gunderson JG, Links PS. Borderline personality disorder: a clinical guide. Arlington, VA: American Psychiatric Publishing; 2008.
4. Ovesiew F, Munich R. Principles of inpatient psychiatry. Philadelphia, PA: Lippincott, Williams and Wilkins; 2009.
5. Main T. The ailment. Br J Med Psychol. 1957;30(3):129–45.

6. Weinberg I, Ronningstam E, Goldblatt MJ, Schechter M, Maltsberger JT. Common factors in empirically supported treatments of borderline personality disorder. Curr Psychiatr Rep. 2011;13(1):60–8.

7. Yeomans FE, Clarkin JF, Kernberg OF. Transference-focused psychotherapy for borderline personality disorder: a clinical guide. 1st ed. Washington, DC: American Psychiatric Publishing; 2015.

8. Zerbo E, Cohen S, Bielska W, Caligor E. Transference-focused psychotherapy in the general psychiatry residency: a useful and applicable model for residents in acute clinical settings. Psychodyn Psychiatry. 2013;41(1):163–81.

9. Bernstein J, Zimmerman M, Auchincloss E. Transference-focused psychotherapy training during residency: an aide to learning psychodynamic psychotherapy. Psychodyn Psychiatry. 2015;43(2):201–22.

10. Paris J. Is hospitalization useful for suicidal patients with borderline personality disorder? J Pers Disord. 2004;18(3):240–7.

11. Bland AR, Rossen EK. Clinical supervision of nurses working with patients with borderline personality disorder. Issues Ment Health Nurs. 2005;26(5):507–17.

12. Lieb K, Zanarini MC, Schmahl C, Linehan MM, Bohus M. Borderline personality disorder. Lancet. 2004;364:453–61.

13. Zanarini MC, Frankenburg FR, Khera GS, Bleichmar J. Treatment histories of borderline patients. Compr Psychiatr. 2001;42(2):144–50.

14. Zanarini MC, Frankenburg FR, Reich DB, Harned AL, Fitzmaurice GM. Rates of psychotropic medication use reported by borderline patients and axis II comparison subjects over 16 years of prospective follow-up. J Clin Psychopharmacol. 2015;35(1):63–7.

15. Lieb K, Vollm B, Rucker G, Timmer A, Stoffers JM. Pharmacotherapy for borderline personality disorder: cochrane systematic review of randomised trials. Br J Psychiatr. 2010;196(1):4–12.

Chapter 6
Transference-Focused Psychotherapy (TFP) Principles in the Pharmacotherapy of Personality Disorders

1. *Using the structural interview broadens the diagnostic process for prescribers.*
2. *Disclosure and psychoeducation serve as critical elements in the pharmacologic treatment of patients with personality disorders.*
3. *TFP principles support a focus on the treatment frame in prescribing in light of any aspects of significant personality pathology revealed in the assessment process.*
4. *TFP principles stress creating a safe environment for the patient and the prescriber.*
5. *TFP principles stress engaging patients in an explicit discussion of treatment goals for pharmacotherapy.*
6. *Using TFP principles to manage affect storms related to medications.*
7. *Managing split treatments in a variety of settings using TFP principles.*

© Springer International Publishing Switzerland 2016
R.G. Hersh et al., *Fundamentals of Transference-Focused Psychotherapy*, DOI 10.1007/978-3-319-44091-0_6

6.1   Introduction

Prescribing medication to patients with personality disorder diagnoses can be challenging and confusing [1]. Patients with some personality disorder diagnoses, particularly borderline personality disorder (BPD), use a lot of medications even though evidence for the effectiveness of these medications is limited [2]. Using transference-focused psychotherapy (TFP) principles can be of help to prescribing clinicians even if these clinicians do not plan to engage in psychotherapy with these patients [3, 4]. TFP principles can help clinicians with the process of comprehensive diagnostic assessment, with creation of an environment ensuring both patients and prescribers feel safe, and with management of patient expectations and patient response to medication trials.

The clinician prescribing psychotropic medications to a patient with either a primary personality disorder or some other psychiatric disorder and co-occurring personality disorder is faced with limited and at times conflicting data. No medication has ever been approved by the Food and Drug Administration for the treatment of personality disorder symptoms. The studies available, for the most part focused on pharmacotherapy of BPD, suggest patients will have limited responses to medication, if at all [5]. While the American Psychiatric Association Guideline for the Treatment of Patients with Borderline Personality Disorder offers what could be seen as a reliable algorithm, the section on medication recommendations has been controversial from its inception [6, 7]. In addition, rigorous evaluations such as the Cochrane Review give only tepid endorsement of pharmacotherapy for most patients with personality disorders, and the United Kingdom's NICE guideline suggests avoiding medication for borderline personality altogether if possible [8, 9].

The literature on pharmacotherapy of personality disorders is disproportionately focused on the treatments of patients with BPD. This discussion is largely informed by that literature, with the goal of extending TFP principles in prescribing beyond patients with BPD to other patients with moderate to severe personality disorder pathology. The structural interview focuses on the elucidation of the patient's level of personality organization by active exploration of identity consolidation (vs. diffusion), nature of defenses employed (repression- vs. splitting-based), and reality testing, among other areas of investigation. Almost all patients with BPD are therefore understood as having moderate to severe personality disorder pathology, as are patients with other DSM-5 diagnoses including paranoid and schizoid personality disorders. The structural interview also explores diagnoses not described in the DSM-5 including hypochondriacal, hypomanic, and sadomasochistic personality disorders. Some, but not all, patients with narcissistic personality disorder will be understood as having moderate to severe pathology. The principles in prescribing to this broader group of patients will differ from practice in prescribing to those patients with a neurotic level of organization, and those patients with a psychotic level of organization including patients with chronic psychotic illness.

Therefore, prescribing clinicians treating patients with significant personality disorder pathology may be faced with the following: symptomatic patients (sometimes suicidal), often high rates of phamacotherapy, limited data (almost all of it short-term, while patients take psychiatric medications for years, if not decades), and contradictory recommendations from various authoritative bodies.

6.2 Using the Structural Interview to Broaden the Diagnostic Process

- *The prescribing clinician has to distinguish between the patient's chief complaint (what the patient reports and the diagnoses he/she believes are relevant) and the clinician's differential diagnosis (what the clinician believes the relevant diagnoses to be).*

(continued)

(continued)

- *The structural interview compels the clinician to think beyond certain limited diagnostic categories.*
- *The clinician can use the diagnostic assessment to prepare for what is to come in the treatment.*
- *The clinician can use the diagnostic assessment to begin to weigh potential benefits and limits of medication.*
- *The structural interview, given its comprehensive approach and use of clarification and confrontation, implicitly challenges a frequent patient-prescriber dyad: "You and your medications have a magic that alone are enough to fix me."*

TFP offers clinicians a systematic approach to pharmacotherapy, beginning with use of the structural interview as part of the diagnostic process. The structural interview compels the clinician to think about the patient's psychological structures that underlie functioning and may reflect personality pathology.

Patients will present to prescribers with particular symptoms and often with an idea of what the diagnosis might be. The prescriber might accept the patient's (or other clinician's) diagnostic formulation at face value. The structural interview, however, requires the prescriber to approach the patient's current symptoms and history systematically beyond the diagnoses offered by the patient and other treaters. This can sometimes cause friction in an initial evaluation as the patient may assume that a chief complaint/established diagnosis ("I have attention deficit disorder" or "I'm here for treatment for my major depression") should be unquestioningly accepted by the clinician as the patient's working diagnosis.

The information obtained in the structural interview allows the clinician to conceptualize the patient's presenting concerns in two critical ways. First, the clinician can make diagnoses consistent with the DSM-5 descriptive categories.

Second, the clinician can begin to speculate about the patient's underlying psychic structure not necessarily captured in DSM-5 nosology, informing initial consideration about the treatments and frame best suited for the presenting problems.

The structural interview differs from a standard "decision-tree" approach to assessment and diagnosis; it is more "freewheeling" in its approach, "circular" meaning the interviewer repeatedly circles back to probe areas of confusion or conflict, generally more broadly curious about areas of functioning often overlooked or given short shrift in an abbreviated "social history" questioning.

The structural interview will give the prescribing clinician a way to think about and describe the patient routinely dismissed with an unspecified personality disorder diagnosis by describing the patient's level of organization. The patient meeting DSM-5 criteria (five of nine criteria for BPD or NPD) will be captured in the structural interview, but so, too, will a significant number of patients who may have subsyndromal presentations (e.g., four of nine BPD criteria or fewer) or, say, narcissistic personality disorder symptoms better described as "vulnerable" or "thin-skinned" and not necessarily captured using the DSM-5 criteria [10].

The prescriber beginning treatment with the structural interview will be better able to engage a patient in the informed consent process. The prescriber will have a clearer sense of the symptoms that are likely to be addressed effectively with medication and those that are not. The prescriber will also be alert to emerging dyads in the patient-prescriber relationship that could impact the patient's response to medication. For example, the patient experiencing herself as needy and the prescriber as powerful may have an initial, intense but short-lived positive response to a treatment. Another possible dyad could be a threatened patient experiencing the prescriber as aggressive, leading to an immediate, negative response to any particular intervention.

The prescriber may choose to use some version of the structural interview with its deliberate and systematic investigation of the patient's understanding of his/her complaints, history, and object relations. While this process (often more involved or confrontational than a standard medical model interview) may cause the patient to feel frustrated or impatient, it will automatically address one particular patient-prescriber dyad often seen in patients with serious personality disorder pathology: powerless patient seeking help from idealized prescribing clinician. The patient's response to the interview can serve as a valuable, early window into the patient's internal world.

Dr. H. Requires Ms. P. to Participate in a Comprehensive Evaluation Prior to Prescribing Medication, Much to the Patient's Dismay

Clinical vignette: Ms. P., a college senior, is referred to Dr. H. (a psychiatrist) by her internist for an evaluation of possible depressive disorder symptoms. Ms. P. had conveyed to her internist recent suicidal thoughts and unstable mood. Dr. H. begins by reviewing with Ms. P. the symptoms she had conveyed to her internist and takes a full inventory of depression symptoms including neurovegetative symptoms. Dr. H. also questions Ms. P. about other areas of her life with the goal of learning about her degree of identity consolidation, her level of defensive functioning, and her reality testing.

Ms. P. becomes irritated during the interview: "I came here for medication for my depression and you're asking me all these questions about my friends and my studies!"

Dr. H. responds: "I want to get a full picture of what is going on with you now. The more I understand about you, your functioning, and your social life, among other things, the more clear I can be without about how medication can and cannot be of help to you." While Ms. P. remains

(continued)

(continued)

irritated for the remainder of the evaluation, Dr. H. senses he has quickly learned about important elements of Ms. P.'s object relations in this process. In particular, Dr. H. is struck by Ms. P.'s reflexive distrust of him and her wariness about his interest in the details of her life. He notes that Ms. P. ascribes to him a malevolent intrusiveness, which seems important given the few details he has learned about the sources of her mood disturbance, including arguments with her roommates and conflict with her department chair about fulfilling the requirements for graduation. Dr. H. feels more prepared for the likely course of Ms. P.'s treatment, knowing something about her experiences with others and having witnessed during their intake together important details for her experience of him.

Take Home Point: Clinicians will benefit from conducting a comprehensive evaluation before prescribing medication and in doing so can quickly learn valuable information about the patient's level of organization and object relations.

6.3 Using Disclosure and Psychoeducation as Part of Effective Prescribing

- *The clinician sets an example of being honest and forthright.*
- *The clinician prepares the patient (and family) and himself/herself for what may happen in the treatment.*
- *The clinician can guide the patient to evidence-based treatments.*

(continued)

(continued)

- *The clinician can guide the patient away from ineffective or even damaging treatments.*
- *The clinician protects himself/herself through effective risk management.*

Comprehensive diagnosis facilitates first discussion with a patient about a clinician's impression, coupled with psychoeducation, and then establishment of a treatment frame. Clinical experience suggests that many patients with personality disorders or personality disorder traits are not aware of their diagnoses [11]. While all of the evidence-based treatments for borderline personality disorder include frank discussion of the borderline diagnosis in their manualized treatment, many clinicians remain reluctant to do so [12]. In particular, prescribing clinicians may see their role as relatively narrow and feel discussion of personality disorder symptoms, in general, as appropriate only for clinicians in the psychotherapist role.

The TFP approach includes attention to the safety and security of the clinician as well as the patient. For the clinician treating a patient with moderate to severe personality disorder symptoms, honest and open discussion with the patient, psychoeducation for the family, and clear documentation about the contribution of personality disorder symptoms are all key elements of both good clinical care and proactive medicolegal self-protection [13].

Families of patients with personality disorder symptoms are often confused when patients do not improve when receiving standard treatments for the mood, anxiety, or other diagnoses that they believe are the primary diagnoses. Clinicians can put themselves in a bind when they are thinking in terms of and documenting one diagnosis (a personality disorder) but conveying to the patient and family only other diagnoses (depression, anxiety, attention disorders). Patients now routinely seek access to their charts (consistent with HIPAA regulations) and may discover that the clinician has been describing personality disorder symptoms in the chart but withholding this information from them, sometimes over many years.

Honest discussion with patients and families about personality disorder diagnoses allows the clinician to guide the patient to evidence-based treatments and to help them avoid those treatments unlikely to be of help or associated with risks of concerning side effects. Clinicians may be fearful that discussion of personality disorder diagnoses will lead a patient to become angry or suicidal. Investigation of the outcome of borderline personality disorder diagnosis disclosure has underscored that, in fact, many patients are relieved to be told they have a well-described and treatable condition, often after going for years feeling they have some form of "treatment-resistant" pathology [14].

The prescribing clinician making a personality disorder diagnosis can use DSM-5 terminology in discussion with some patients. Many clinicians are increasingly comfortable speaking frankly with patients about borderline personality disorder, given growing research about the disorder's generally positive prognosis and multiple evidence-based treatments [15, 16]. The prescriber may choose to review with a patient the DSM-5 BPD criteria as part of a psycho-education intervention [17]. Alternatively, some clinicians may choose to convey their diagnostic impression using their own language for aspects of the disorder. The clinician may say, "You've been describing ways that fluctuations in your self-esteem can cause you difficulties," rather than use the term narcissistic personality disorder, or with a patient with BPD traits, "What you describe as brief periods of 'depression' when in conflict with friends and family sounds more like mood instability and reactivity than the persistent low mood we would expect to see with major depression."

TFP-informed psychotherapy stresses that the clinician cannot be optimally helpful to the patient when feeling anxious and unsafe. The prescriber aware that a patient has personality disorder symptoms but uncomfortable discussing this observation puts himself or herself in a compromising position. The personality disorder symptoms remain "the elephant in the room," and breaking the silence about these symptoms can help the clinician practice in a more honest and less anxious fashion.

Ms. B. Presents to the Nurse Practitioner for Medications for "Depression"

Clinical vignette: Ms. B. is an attorney in her late 20s who has been receiving care for "treatment-resistant depression" for many years. She has become increasingly frustrated as she has failed to respond to a variety of antidepressant medications and most recently has gained 30 pounds from an adjunctive antipsychotic medication, which has failed to address her pattern of suicidal despair with every breakup with her fiancé. Ms. B. moves to a new city and transfers her care to a nurse practitioner, Mr. Z. Mr. Z. tells Ms. B. he would like a chance to review her history and spend a few sessions getting to know her before making any conclusions about her diagnosis or treatment options.

Ms. B. recounts for Mr. Z. her history of multiple medication trials. Ms. B. also describes her referral to a dialectical behavior therapy-informed mindfulness group; she notes that she attended the group sporadically and tells Mr. Z. she cannot recall any discussion of personality disorders as part of the group discussion.

After three sessions Mr. Z. feels comfortable introducing to Ms. B. the idea that she likely has a primary or co-occurring personality disorder with borderline traits. This diagnosis comes as a suprise to Ms. B., who had assumed her condition was a "treatment-resistant

(continued)

(continued)

depression." Mr. Z. takes the opportunity to review the borderline personality disorder diagnostic criteria and the best available evidence about the effectiveness of various medications and psychotherapies. He also invites Ms. B.'s fiancé to come to a session to discuss these issues. While Ms. B. is initially confused and angry when Mr. Z. shares his impressions, she recovers quickly and reflects: "I always wondered why I was never getting better. Something just didn't fit, and this diagnosis, as difficult as it is, explains a lot of things for me."

Take Home Point: While a patient with personality disorder symptoms may present to a clinician specifically for treatment with medication, the clinician should feel comfortable educating the patient about the centrality of psychotherapy in the treatment of personality disorders and the relative limits of pharmacotherapy.

6.4   Introduction of the Treatment Frame in Prescribing

- *Prescribers often work without a clearly defined treatment frame.*
- *Patients with moderate to severe personality disorder pathology will predictably challenge the prescriber's routine way of working.*
- *Working with patients with impulsivity, suicidality, or non-adherence will require a thoroughly considered treatment frame.*
- *Prescribing medications toxic in overdose requires increased attention to the treatment frame.*
- *Prescribing medications requiring vigilance about adherence or associated necessary laboratory testing requires increased attention to the treatment frame.*

In TFP the contracting phase is integrated into the establishment of a treatment frame. The frame allows the patient's object relations pathology to unfold in a way that is safe and controlled for both the patient and the therapist. The TFP therapist engages the patient, even before the treatment begins, to consider what likely treatment-interfering behaviors might emerge. In general, the TFP approach (for psychotherapy) follows the dictum that the more symptomatic the patient, the more rigorous the frame.

The prescribing clinician accustomed to a medical model approach with patients may not have treatment frame concerns in mind at the beginning of a treatment. The clinician actively considering primary or co-occurring personality disorder symptoms should be stimulated to engage the patient in a detailed discussion of the treatment frame even when the patient and the prescriber are not engaged in concurrent psychotherapy.

The TFP understanding of the borderline patient's object relations will stimulate the clinician to expect certain prescriber-clinician dyads to emerge. The patient may see herself as vulnerable and powerless and expect the prescriber to be magically effective; another expectable dyad could be the patient who feels poorly cared for and continually at risk for harm from the careless psychiatrist's damaging medications.

A focus on the treatment frame can address some of these predictable patient-prescriber dyads and their associated complications. An example is the patient who has a rapidly shifting experience of the clinician from highly idealized ("This doctor's medications are certain to make me feel better") to persecutory ("These medications are making me worse and I have to stop them myself"). In a case like this, the clinician may in advance predict for the patient the possibility of a shift like this and underscore a need for the patient to make decisions about medications in consultation with the prescriber and not independently or abruptly.

How else can discussion of the treatment frame be of use? The treatment frame should include a clear discussion of basic logistical issues (payment, missed session policies, lateness) as well as those issues often pertinent with patients with moderate to severe personality disorder symptomatology (non-adherence, dishonesty, suicidality, threats of violence). The prescriber should, at the outset, review explicitly with the patient the requirements for continued treatment. While this might not be routine management, the prescriber attuned to severe personality disorder pathology will predict challenges by the patient to the clinician's standard practice patterns.

Many patients with significant personality disorder symptoms will be prescribed medications with concerning side effects. Medications toxic in overdose (lithium carbonate, tricyclic antidepressants), with dietary restrictions (monoamine oxidase inhibitors), or requiring periodic laboratory testing (atypical antipsychotics), can present particular problems to the prescriber. The clinician aware in advance of a patient's personality disorder symptoms can predict probable complications given an understanding of likely dominant dyads in the transference and associated reversals.

In TFP the therapist will review with patients specific treatment-threatening behaviors that will likely preclude an effective psychotherapy process. The therapist will be clear about the futility of TFP when a patient is frequently hospitalized, or severely underweight, or actively using drugs and alcohol in a way that compromises the patient's capacity to use the treatment. The prescriber is likewise helped by establishing a clear frame at the outset of treatment, with attention to behaviors that would interrupt the potential success of medication trials. Explicit discussion of issues like non-adherence, misuse of medication, or requirements for specific laboratory testing at the beginning of treatment can help the clinician manage expected situations that arise challenging the frame that is already clearly in place.

Ms. G. Refused to Get the Blood Tests Required for
Treatment with Lithium

Clinical vignette: Mrs. G. was hospitalized three times in 2
months with recurrent suicidality. She was diagnosed with
borderline personality disorder and narcissistic personality
disorder traits by the inpatient team. The inpatient team had
doubts about Mrs. G.'s prior diagnosis of bipolar disorder,
Type II, but nevertheless continued her lithium carbonate
during her hospitalizations. In the past Mrs. G. would follow
a pattern of ignoring her prescriber's recommendations for
follow-up testing of the lithium carbonate level. Mrs. G.'s
response to her prescribers had alternated between periods
of idealization ("Finally a doctor who understands my
mood disorder and is going to do something about it!")
with persecutory feelings ("Haven't I been stuck enough for
blood tests! You want me to get another lithium level so you
feel better, but I'm the one who ends up bruised and for no
reason, because I can tell my level is fine!").

Mrs. G.'s inpatient psychiatrist, Dr. L., agrees to work
with her after discharge but with certain conditions.
Aware of Mrs. G.'s personality disorder symptoms and
pattern of impulsivity, Dr. L. tells Mrs. G. she is not willing
to prescribe lithium to her at this time and reviews which
medications she would be comfortable prescribing (a
mood stabilizer not toxic in overdose) and what her limits
would be should Mrs. G. not adhere to her recommenda-
tions (periodic screening for metabolic syndrome if she
chooses to continue on an atypical antipsychotic medica-
tion). Mrs. G. protests and states flatly she will "stay on
lithium and never give a blood sample again!" Dr. L.
meets with Mrs. G. and her husband and informs them
she will help find another prescriber for Mrs. G.'s outpatient
treatment as she is not willing to work with her without a
mutually agreed-upon frame in place.

Take Home Point: The prescriber should establish a
treatment frame that insures safety for both the patient
and clinician.

6.5 Creating a Safe Environment for the Patient and the Prescriber

- *Psychoeducation about the limited effectiveness of pharmacotherapy for personality disorders, and certain co-occurring conditions (e.g., depression, anxiety) when personality disorder symptomatology is present, will protect the clinician.*
- *Departure from standard practices should trigger exploration of countertransference.*
- *Departures, including supplying patients with unusually large amounts of medication or prescribing doses about those recommended by FDA guidelines, should be "red flags."*
- *Monitoring of polypharmacy with clear communication about the overarching goal of using as little medication as possible is imperative.*

TFP emphasizes the need for a clear treatment framework and associated contract with a goal of creating a safe environment for the patient and therapist. Without a safe environment, the therapist cannot stay focused on the patient in a helpful way. An appreciation of the patient's level of organization helps the prescribing clinician put into place a treatment frame that will best insure safety and security for both the patient and the clinician. Some of these issues are concrete: Should the clinician give a patient likely to be impulsive a medication toxic in overdose? Should a clinician adjust a complex medication regimen for a patient likely to be compliant only with the simplest instructions? How does the prescriber manage a patient who might be dishonest and feigning symptoms to get medication? The treatment frame includes concerns as mentioned (supplies of medication, complexity of the regimen) as well as other nuts-and-bolts concerns (e.g., the necessity of communication with other

clinicians, communication with family if needed, requirements for certain laboratory testing), and frank discussions
about potentially interfering behaviors (substance use, eating
disorders) that could undermine the effectiveness of a medication trial.

The TFP approach can protect the prescriber in a number
of ways. Explicit discussion of the limits of medication in the
treatment of personality disorders (and in the treatment of
co-occurring conditions for patients with personality disorders) is imperative and prepares the patient and family for
equivocal results. This helps clinicians avoid a number of
problematic situations. In one common scenario, patients and
families become angry because of the failure of standard
treatments for putative mood, anxiety, or other disorders. In
another situation often seen, clinicians may feel compelled to
use unusual medication combinations or above-recommended
medication doses for patients unresponsive to routine medications at recommended doses.

The TFP focus on monitoring countertransference can aid
clinicians who might put themselves at risk when prescribing
for patients with personality disorders. The clinician will
reflect: Am I departing from my standard practices? What
may be happening with this patient to cause me to do things
I would not ordinarily do? The clinician poised to prescribe
more medication than usual, to use medications off-label in
uncomfortable-making ways, or to combine medications in
counterintuitive ways, will automatically speculate about the
transference-countertransference meanings of these actions.

Patients with BPD are known to be high utilizers of medications in all categories, often leading to complex polypharmacy [18]. There is no data supporting the practice of
polypharmacy with patients with personality disorders. This
polypharmacy puts patients at risk for drug-drug interactions
of all kinds. The clinician focused on creating a safe environment will be compelled to address habitual polypharmacy
through both psychoeducation and prescribing practices.
This process is aided by awareness of likely dyads and their
reversals. For example, the prescriber feeling pressured to
add a medication to a patient in crisis may reflect on both the

patient-prescriber dyad of vulnerable patient seeking help from the powerful clinician and its reversal of aggressive patient demanding action from a cowed clinician.

Ms. D.'s Weight Loss Frightens the Resident Assigned to Manage Her Medications

Clinical vignette: Dr. B. is a psychiatry resident working in a clinic for trainees. She is assigned to work with Ms. D., a 29-year-old unemployed woman with borderline personality disorder. The resident turning over responsibility for Ms. D.'s care described his longstanding anxiety treating Ms. D., given the patient's pattern of restricting her intake at times leading to a marked decrease in her weight to a body mass index of 16 (severely underweight).

Dr. B. learns that the previous resident was so anxious with every visit and so preoccupied with Ms. D.'s weight that it was hard for him to concentrate in the sessions, imagining that Ms. D. would develop a cardiac arrhythmia and die while taking the antidepressant medication he had prescribed. Dr. B.'s TFP training reinforced the necessity of a safe environment for both the patient and clinician. Dr. B. was also aware of the oscillating dyad of weak, vulnerable patient fearful of withholding prescriber and persistently uncomfortable prescriber controlled by the patient manipulating her dangerously low weight.

Dr. B. therefore resolved to set a specific weight threshold for the patient and insisted on ongoing contact with the patient's internist. The patient responded with tearful indignation, which had been her pattern with the previous trainee. Dr. B. was aware of her temptation to accomodate this patient but had held fast, knowing she would not be able to think clearly in the kind of anxiety-producing setting Ms. D. had been engendering.

Take Home Point: The prescriber should use her countertransference to determine the requirements for a treatment frame that would allow her treat her patient without undue anxiety.

6.6   Explicit Discussion of Goals for Medication as an Essential Part of Treatment

- *Clinicians may not explicitly convey to patients medications' adjunctive role.*
- *Patients may assume that medications alone will address personality disorder symptoms.*
- *Personality disorder patients are often started on medications during crises.*
- *Personality disorder patients often continue on medications without periodic reviews of their effectiveness.*
- *Discussion of goals for medication helps patients take responsibility for those symptoms not likely to improve with medication alone.*

TFP requires an explicit discussion of treatment goals as part of the contracting phase of the psychotherapy. Discussion of goals can help the therapist avoid extended, aimless treatments that can inadvertently contribute to a patient's passivity. Along these lines the prescribing clinician using TFP principles will focus on goals for pharmacotherapy when any new agent is introduced and then again with every meeting. This emphasis on an explicit discussion of treatment goals helps clinicians avoid the common pitfalls associated with complex and unwieldy polypharmacy (a widely described hallmark of medicating patients with personality disorders). The discussion of goals also underscores the expectation in TFP that treatment is not static but built on an expectation that patients will change over time.

Explicit discussion of goals for medication for patients with personality disorder diagnoses begins with a discussion of the likely *adjunctive* role of medication in their treatment. This proviso is strongly supported by the literature. Discussion of medication's adjunctive role also directly addresses a common patient-prescriber dyad: "You and your medications alone are enough to fix me!" More complicated are those patients with both mood or anxiety (or other) disorders with co-occurring personality disorder symptoms. Again, the literature underscores the likelihood that medications effective for the mood or anxiety disorder alone are less effective for those conditions in patients with co-occurring personality disorder symptoms [19].

Discussion of medication goals directly addresses a common pattern seen in psychotherapy with patients with personality disorders, specifically a passivity suggesting an unconscious expectation that the treater alone can fix the patient's problems. The patient with personality disorder symptoms telling the prescriber "I just want these medications to make me happier!" will benefit from a discussion of how medication can help (targeting specific symptoms) and how they cannot (addressing underlying object relations/patterns of experiencing self and others associated with chronic discontent or self-defeating behaviors).

Patients presenting in crisis may demand relief with medications. TFP principles prepare clinicians to monitor their countertransference in such situations, rather than act impulsively themselves. The complying prescriber responding in a crisis may then find the patient experiences any attempt in the future to remove a medication as depriving or even damaging. The prescriber managing a patient in crisis can help avoid the common pitfall of adding yet another medication and renewing it routinely by articulating a specific plan in advance. Such a plan would include the intention to stop a medication within a specific period of time if it is not working or after a particular crisis has resolved. Even medications begun routinely should be reevaluated periodically with a stated overarching goal of using as little medication as possible. Many patients and prescribers can drift into a custodial relationship, thus engaging in a mutual enactment that confirms through inaction the patient's unconscious object relation of the incapacitated patient and indifferent clinician.

Ms. D. Has a Complicated Medication Regimen that Does Not Seem to Be Helping

Clinical vignette: Ms. D. presents to Dr. R. for an evaluation after she has a suicide attempt by overdose in the context of chronic conflict with her wife. Ms. D. was seen periodically by a prescriber who saw her in a high-volume clinic for 15 minutes every other month. Ms. D. was under the impression she had attention deficit disorder, obsessive compulsive disorder, and depression and anxiety symptoms.

On presentation to Dr. R., Ms. D. was taking an antidepressant medication, two stimulants, a benzodiazepine, and a mood stabilizer. Dr. R. speaks with the prior treater who agrees that Ms. D. likely has moderate to severe narcissistic personality disorder (NPD) traits which are predominantly responsible for her chronic distress in her marriage and recent suicidality.

After an extended evaluation, Dr. R. reviews with Ms. D. his tentative diagnostic impression, using layman's terms, stressing the typical pattern of highly variable self-esteem seen in patients with NPD. He also proposes a systematic paring of the patient's medication regimen with the goal of removing possible confounding side effects and focusing on exploration of long-standing personality rigidity related to marked fluctuations in her self-esteem. Ms. D. responds affirmatively to Dr. R.'s initial explanation of his diagnostic impression, asking "When you say ups and downs of self-esteem, and sensitivity to injury, do you mean narcissistic traits?" Dr. R. responds, "Now that you mention it, yes, I think that captures a lot of what you have described." Ms. D. is initially uncomfortable with the proposal to reduce her medications, describing an apprehension that Dr. R. is depriving her of sources of symptom relief. On further questioning Ms. D. is unable to ascribe any particular

(continued)

(continued)

symptom relief to any specific medication but acknowledges having had a sense that her prior prescriber "cared" for her as evidenced by his willingness to prescribe a new medication with almost every visit. Dr. H. proposes first stopping the mood stabilizer, in part because of its apparent sedating property, and then stopping one or both of the stimulants that had been used, in part, to counteract the sedation from the mood stabilizer. Dr. H. suggests that a regimen of an antidepressant and a benzodiazepine taken as needed might be adequate for Ms. D. Ms. D. reluctantly agrees to go forward with this plan.

Take Home Point: The clinician prescribing medication to the patient with significant personality disorder symptoms should periodically engage the patient in a detailed discussion of the goals for use of any medication.

6.7   Managing Affect Storms

- *Patients' affect storms are predictable but still unnerving for the prescriber.*
- *TFP can provide an overarching way of understanding affect storms and helpful ways for clinicians to manage these episodes.*
- *Effective management in an affect storm can be containing and, in time, foster the patient-clinician relationship.*

Prescribing clinicians may often become aware of a patient's use of splitting-based defenses in the context of a patient's "affect storm." A typical scenario would be a patient's rapid shift from an idealizing to an intensely devaluing experience of the prescriber. A patient's heightened emotional state seen in an affect storm often includes powerful elements of anger or fear. The unsuspecting clinician can easily become fearful or angry or disengaged in such a context, often leading to decision-making about prescribing hampered by these reactions. An understanding of the underlying object relations predisposing patients to heightened affective states can help guide clinicians during periods when an unsuspecting clinician may be likely to act rashly in response.

TFP psychotherapists will use the technique of "naming the actors" in situations when they feel overwhelmed, which is not uncommon with patients with severe personality disorders. "Naming the actors" helps the clinician begin to describe the dominant object relations dyad (and thereby orienting the clinician during a period of confusion), and at the same time these comments can help contain a patient by showing the patient that the clinician has an understanding of the patient's subjective experience (and sometimes helping the patient put the intense experience into words).

In an affect storm the patient will be overwhelmed by feelings to the point of becoming unable to think clearly. Often the affect storm will feature powerful paranoid feelings, with prominent suspicion, anger, or even threats toward the clinician. In TFP the affect storm is often managed by the clinician by a shift to "therapist-centered interpretations." In this model, the clinician aware of the patient's heightened affective state and compromised capacity to think clearly will articulate how the clinician believes the patient is experiencing him or her in the moment.

The prescriber using TFP principles will approach the patient in a heightened affective state with a strategy as how best to proceed. The prescriber will know to avoid defensive arguments ("You're angry with me, but I was clear with you from the start about this side effect") or interpretations ("You're angry with me the way you describe feeling angry with your father when he ignored you"). Instead the prescriber will focus on containing the affect ("You are experiencing me now as threatening and depriving") and, if possible, on the role reversal ("You accused me of threatening you by refusing to renew your Klonopin given your recent alcohol binge, while addressing me in a way that has a somewhat threatening quality, as if you are about to throw your coffee at me.")

Clinicians may be surprised by a patient's "affect storm," particularly internists or family physicians with limited experience treating patients with severe personality disorders. Often the patient's "affect storm" is the first occasion when an unsuspecting clinician grasps the likely object relations underneath the patient's intense anger and devaluation.

Mr. L. Explodes at His Internist, Causing Turmoil in the Office

Clinical vignette: Mr. L., a professional dancer with borderline personality disorder, begins his appointment with his internist, who prescribes his psychiatric medications, in a heightened state of distress. Mr. L. is visibly angry as he enters Dr. Y.'s office: "I can't believe my mother didn't call your front desk with my new insurance information! I'll have to pay out of pocket for everything and I'll be broke!" Dr. Y. was familiar with Mr. L.'s history of intense anger and recurrent pattern of feeling poorly cared for by those he depended on. While Dr. Y. was familiar with the diagnosis of borderline personality disorder, he had only recently been exposed to TFP principles in managing patients.

Initially Dr. Y.'s secretary attempted to defend the office, which only increased Mr. L.'s level of anger. Dr. Y. brought Mr. L. into his office and, aware of his diagnosis and oriented to use TFP principles, Dr. Y. made an effort to avoid becoming defensive and instead tried to contain Mr. L. by putting into words Mr. L.'s feelings of being

(continued)

(continued)

poorly care for: "You feel as if I am indifferent and our office uncaring about you and your finances." Mr. L. calmed a bit and Dr. Y. continued: "You were feeling mistreated by your mother and our office, at the same time you were yelling at my office manager and causing her to feel mistreated." Mr. L. was able to recover enough to begin to think clearly; he and Dr. Y. were able to complete their visit as planned.

Take Home Point: All prescribers of psychiatric medications can use TFP interventions to manage patients who become "difficult" because of heightened affective states and poor coping strategies.

6.8   Managing Split Treatments

- *The TFP focus on the patient's splitting-based defenses predicts splitting behavior in divided treatment.*
- *The prescribing clinician, expecting problematic splitting in divided treatment, will set up protections in the treatment contract.*
- *Protections can include requirement of permission to speak to the therapist, other involved clinicians, and family members.*
- *The TFP clinician can expect problematic splitting when the patient interfaces with other settings such as emergency rooms or inpatient units.*

Prescribing clinicians will see personality disordered patients in a number of settings. In recent years, for a variety of reasons, the prescribing psychiatrist is more likely than in the past to work with another clinician who assumes responsibility for providing psychotherapy [20]. Managing split treatments, while at times challenging with many patients, is inevitably challenging with patients with serious personality disorders. The expected pattern of alternating idealizing and devaluing one or both of the clinicians involved can create particularly thorny situations. TFP principles can help guide clinicians, both prescriber and psychotherapist, using object relations theory to explain what clinicians are accustomed to encountering in practice. Both/all parties involved in the care of the patient should be aware that a patient with borderline psychological structure seeks a perfect level of caretaking that is considered impossible and that anything that falls short of it may be seen as neglect or mistreatment.

The prescriber will need to be alert to any number of concerning situations. For example, the patient referred by a longtime therapist to a psychiatrist for evaluation may experience the prescriber in a wholly negative way, which may cause the therapist to collude with the patient's devaluation of the option of medication. Also concerning would be the prescriber who devalues a therapist's attempts to maintain the frame, again colluding with the patient's experience of a therapist holding to a frame as arbitrary, rigid, uncaring, or even punitive.

The prescriber cannot safely treat a patient without permission to speak freely with the patient's therapist. The patient's refusal to grant this permission should be grounds to end the treatment. Both parties (prescriber and therapist) should require communication at the outset of any treatment, thereby addressing the predictable emergence of a split between treaters.

Patients with severe personality disorders seen in routine outpatient care may interface with clinicians in other settings such as partial hospital programs, emergency rooms, and inpatient units. Again, the prescriber will be alert to the emergence of splitting in the "team" as patients may use the opportunity of time in a new setting to devalue a long-standing treater while temporarily idealizing a new clinician. Alternatively, a patient sent by a prescriber to an emergency room or inpatient unit may vociferously devalue the new treaters and enlist the longstanding treater to enact a rescue. The TFP contract foretells such a scenario and outlines, in advance, the requirement that a patient (e.g., acutely suicidal and requiring inpatient treatment for safety) agrees to follow the directives of any emergency room or inpatient clinician. The prescriber who uses this TFP principle can, in such a situation, refer back to the treatment contract and avoid potentially destructive conflict between treaters in different settings.

Dr. P. Becomes Embroiled in a "Split" with Ms. C.'s Inpatient Treatment Team

Clinical vignette: Dr. P. works at a day treatment program where he has been prescribing medication for Ms. C., a college student on leave, now attending the program for approximately 3 months. Ms. C. is hospitalized after a threat to hang herself and is treated on the inpatient unit at the large academic medical center housing the day program. After the hospital admission, Dr. P. begins to get calls from Ms. C., from her mother, and from her social worker therapist at the day program about "mistreatment" Ms. C. is receiving on this unit. Dr. P. is initially skeptical about this but then finds himself more exercised after discussing the situation with the therapist who suggests that Dr. P. should "pull strings" to have Ms. C. transferred. Dr. P. becomes aware of his growing anger at the inpatient staff and his impulse to intercede on Ms. C.'s behalf.

Dr. P.'s familiarity with TFP prompts him to take a step back and monitor his reactions to the calls he was receiving. Soon thereafter, Dr. P. is contacted by the inpatient psychiatrist to arrange a conference call about the patient. At this time, Dr. P. begins to consider the possibility of an evolving split forming between the current inpatient team and Ms. C.'s outpatient treaters. During the conference call,

(continued)

(continued)

Dr. P. is struck by the inpatient clinician's reasonable approach to Ms. C.'s care and his understandable caution about giving Ms. C. increased privileges on the unit given her continued threats to harm herself. Dr. P. is aware that he and Ms. C.'s day program therapist were then more confident in presenting to Ms. C., during a meeting on the unit, their impression that the inpatient staff was managing her care in a reasonable way. Ms. C. was initially defiant in reaction to their meeting. In the subsequent days, however, calls from Ms. C. stopped and the staff on the inpatient unit noticed she was engaging with them in a more cooperative way, acknowledging, "I understand I have to be in good enough control so that you can get me back to the day program. I don't like being here, but you're doing your job."

Take Home Point: Clinicians involved in a "split treatment" with a patient with severe personality disorder pathology will need to remain vigilant about the risk of a schism between treaters, and the related dynamics, which can be a detriment to the patient's recovery.

References

1. Silk KR. The process of managing medications in patients with borderline personality disorder. J Psychiatr Pract. 2011;17(5):311–9.
2. Bender DS, Dolan RT, Skodol AE, Sanislow C, Dyck IR, McGlashan TH, Shea MT, Zanarini MC, Oldham JM, Gunderson JG. Treatment utilization by patients with personality disorders. Am J Psychiatr. 2001;158:295–302.
3. Hersh RG. Using transference-focused psychotherapy principles in the pharmacotherapy of patients with severe personality disorders. Psychodyn Psychiatry. 2015;43(2):181–200.

4. Clarkin JF, Yeomans FE, Kernberg OF. Psychotherapy for borderline personality disorder: focusing on object relations. Washington, DC: American Psychiatric Publishing, Inc.; 2010.
5. Feurino L, Silk KR. State of the art in the pharmacologic treatment of borderline personality disorder. Curr Psychiatr Rep. 2011;13(1):69–75.
6. American Psychiatric Association. Practice guideline for the treatment of patients with borderline personality disorder. Am J Psychiatr. 2001;158:1–52.
7. Paris J. Commentary on the American Psychiatric Association guidelines for the treatment of borderline personality disorder: evidence-based psychiatry and the quality of evidence. J Pers Disord. 2002;16(2):130–4.
8. Lieb K, Vollm B, Rucker G, Timmer A, Stoffers H. Pharmacotherapy for borderline personality disorder: Cochrane systematic review of randomised trials. Br J Psychiatry. 2010; 196(1):4–12.
9. National Institute for Health and Clinical Excellence (NICE). Borderline personality disorder, treatment and managements. London: The British Psychologist Society and the Royal College of Psychiatrists; 2009. www.nice.org.uk/cg78.
10. American Psychiatric Association. Diagnostic and statistical manual of mental disorders. 5th ed. Washington DC; 2014.
11. Gunderson JG, Links P. Handbook of good psychiatric management for borderline personality disorder. Arlington, VA: American Psychiatric Association; 2014.
12. Paris J. Why psychiatrists are reluctant to diagnose borderline personality disorder. Psychiatry. 2007;4(1):35–9.
13. Gutheil TG. Medicolegal pitfalls in the treatment of borderline patients. Am J Psychiatr. 1985;142(1):9–14.
14. Zanarini MC, Frankenburg FR. A preliminary, randomized trial of psychoeducation for women with borderline personality disorder. J Pers Disord. 2008;22(3):284–90.
15. Weinberg I, Ronningstam E, Goldblatt M. Common factors in empirically supported treatments of borderline personality disorder. Curr Psych Rep. 2011;12:60–8.
16. Zanarini MC, Frankenburg F, Reich DB. Time to attainment of recovery from borderline personality disorder and stability of recovery: a 10-year prospective follow-up study. Am J Psychiatr. 2010;167:663–7.
17. LeQuesne ER, Hersh RG. Disclosure of a diagnosis of borderline personality disorder. J Psychiatr Pract. 2004;10:170–6.

18. Zanarini M, Frankenburg F, Hennen J, Silk K. Mental health service utilization by borderline personality disorder patients and axis II comparison subjects followed prospectively for 6 year. J Clin Psychiatr. 2004;65(1):28–36.
19. Gunderson JG, Morey LC, McGlashan TH. Major depressive disorder and borderline personality disorder revisited: longitudinal interactions. J Clin Psychiatr. 2004;65:1049–56.
20. Pincus HA, Tanielian TL, Marcus SC, Olfson MA, Zarin DA, Thompson J, Zito JM. Prescribing trends in psychotropic medications. J Am Med Assoc. 1998;279(7):526–31.

Chapter 7
Transference-Focused Psychotherapy (TFP) Principles in the Management of Co-occurring Medical and Personality Disorder Symptoms

1. *TFP principles can provide clinicians with a useful psychodynamically-informed approach to patients in the overlap between medical and personality disorder (PD) symptoms.*
2. *The TFP contract addresses in advance the direct medical complications of BPD (self-injury, binge eating, physical altercations) or any other treatment-interfering medical symptoms.*
3. *The TFP approach aims to minimize iatrogenic contributions to medical complications (weight gain, metabolic syndrome, sedative-hypnotic or stimulant misuse) in the treatment of personality disorders.*
4. *TFP's expectation for change will dictate the therapist's more active approach to health-related lifestyle choices.*
5. *The TFP approach directly addresses the risk of chronic medical disability as an expression of passivity or parasitism.*

(continued)

© Springer International Publishing Switzerland 2016   187
R.G. Hersh et al., *Fundamentals of Transference-Focused Psychotherapy*, DOI 10.1007/978-3-319-44091-0_7

(continued)

6. *Medical professionals can utilize TFP techniques in their treatment of PD patients without necessarily assuming responsibility for their psychiatric care.*
7. *Medical professionals can utilize TFP techniques and principles with patients who have difficulty with treatment adherence even in the absence of a diagnosable personality disorder.*

7.1   Introduction

Clinicians of all kinds treating patients with personality disorder (PD) pathology find the overlap of medical concerns, and PD symptomatology presents unusually vexing and complex challenges [1]. The goal of this chapter is to extend certain principles informing individual TFP to a variety of situations involving patients with physical complaints and medical problems.

The interface between medical complaints and personality disorder pathology is a daunting subject. The clinical presentations reflecting this interface are highly variable. They can include:

1. Medical sequelae directly related to a personality disorder
2. Medical conditions that have higher than expected rates of comorbidity among PD patients
3. Iatrogenically induced medical issues
4. The effects of poor health-related lifestyle choices
5. Chronic medical syndromes that reflect or reinforce passivity or parasitism
6. Challenges clinicians encounter providing standard medical services to patients with personality disorders and other patients without clear psychiatric diagnoses, but with compromised compliance

In TFP offered as an individual psychotherapy, the assessment and contracting phases take into full account any medical or somatic concerns that might constitute treatment-threatening behavior. The terms "medical" and "somatic" are overlapping but not synonymous. Medical issues can relate to the patient's actual medical diagnoses and treatments, as well as aspects of a patient's general medical care, such as cooperation with an annual physical exam. Somatic symptoms, as distinct from actual medical concerns, might include scenarios such as a heightened sensitivity to medication side effects or limited exercise tolerance because of cigarette smoking – physical concerns that are not necessarily linked to an identifiable medical disorder. In the assessment phase, the therapist will circle back to any medical or somatic symptoms and clarify to what extent the patient has complied with a comprehensive medical assessment process and to what extent the patient has complied with treatment recommendations. The contracting phase has as its goal a thorough investigation of any potentially treatment-interfering behaviors, which could, of course, include medical symptoms precluding full involvement in the treatment or active participation in meaningful work or studies, as is stipulated in the TFP contract. The contracting process leads directly to the establishment and maintenance of the treatment frame; this frame can include patient responsibilities related to somatic or medical concerns.

Iatrogenic complications of treatment for BPD are widely described and remain a serious concern [2]. (See Chap. 6 for a full discussion of a TFP approach to pharmacotherapy.) It is well known that BPD patients are likely to take psychiatric medications at high rates, despite the limited effectiveness of psychoactive medication in the treatment of BPD; research indicates patients with BPD also take *nonpsychiatric* medications at unusually high rates [3]. Iatrogenic complications of misdiagnosis or underdiagnosis of personality disorder pathology can include the medical sequelae of antidepressant, antipsychotic, mood stabilizer, sedative-hypnotic or anxiolytic medications, as well as stimulant abuse or dependence or overuse of narcotic medication for pain [4]. Mental health providers are not the only clinicians involved in iatrogenic complications in the treatment of PD patients; the same dynamics are at work when PD patients interact with clinicians in other branches of medicine. TFP's focus on (1) the active assessment of personality disorder elements and (2) use of contracting to establish a treatment frame can help limit these complications.

TFP departs from other psychoanalytically-informed interventions, including psychoanalysis, by stressing a more active role for the therapist. This more active role may include a focused approach to a patient's health issues and more active confrontation of a patient's poor health-related lifestyle choices. In this case, the TFP therapist might actively confront the apparent contradictions between a patient's stated goals and evidence of poor health-related choices.

TFP is also notable for its particular focus on identifying a passive stance that may favor receipt of care and benefits (the "secondary gain" of illness) in patients with personality disorder pathology. This passive exploitation can sometimes be linked to a patient's somatic or medical concerns. The TFP therapist will be comfortable with an explicit confrontation of a patient's unwillingness to participate in a full medical evaluation or a patient's non-adherence with recommended medical treatment. In the course of treatment, such behavior can be understood as an expression of treatment-interfering behavior or self-destructiveness, to be explored in the context of the transference. The TFP therapist will also be proactive in exploring any medical or somatic concern that might be a factor in a patient's decision to conclude he or she is incapacitated and therefore reliant on family or government for financial support.

While many mental health clinicians have only limited education about personality disorder pathology, it is fair to say that outside of psychiatry, most physicians, physicians' assistants, nurse practitioners, and nurses have had even less. Primary care clinicians from many areas of medicine have gone on record as requesting guidance about how to manage patients with PD symptoms [5, 6]. These clinicians do not necessarily assume responsibility for these patients' psychiatric treatment, but they nonetheless find themselves encountering many of the same issues facing mental health clinicians. TFP interventions useful to psychiatric residents seeing patients in acute care settings (as outlined in Chap. 8), for example, may be similarly useful to primary care clinicians in their own treatment settings [7]. Medical professionals may use TFP principles, including monitoring countertransference, contracting, and identifying dominant dyads and their reversals, when working with patients with primary personality disorder diagnoses or with those patients who simply have difficulty with aspects of compliance.

7.2   A TFP Principle-Based Approach to Managing the Interface Between Medical and Psychiatric Complaints

- *Clinicians can expect varied presentations involving medical and psychiatric complaints in PD patients.*
- *Physical symptoms as a manifestation of personality pathology, and the effect of PD pathology on management of medical self-care, can be overlapping and synergistic.*
- *TFP principles offer a flexible approach to clinical management of medical concerns for clinicians with either primary mental health or medical responsibilities.*
- *TFP principles can help ground clinicians when they face the specific chaos introduced by severe personality pathology.*

The possible combinations of medical or somatic concerns and elements of personality disorder (PD) pathology are many and varied. These combinations will be strikingly familiar to mental health clinicians assuming responsibility for PD patients with medical symptoms and to medical providers charged with providing care to those patients whose treatments are complicated by PD symptoms or simply non-compliance.

The interface between medical and personality disorder pathology can include the following:

- The direct medical consequences of BPD including self-injury (wound care), medical consequences of drug overdoses, obesity related to binge eating, and sequelae to physical altercations
- Medical syndromes identified as having significant rates of comorbidity among PD patients including, among others, fibromyalgia, chronic pain, and obesity
- Iatrogenic complications including side effects of antidepressants (diminished libido, weight gain, akathisia), mood stabilizers (weight gain, sedation), antipsychotic medications (weight gain, metabolic syndrome, akathisia), and anxiolytics, sedative-hypnotics, or stimulants (substance use disorders)
- Poor health-related lifestyle choices (documented in BPD studies) including cigarette smoking, lack of exercise, and daily use of pain medications or sleeping aids
- Medical concerns as central elements in patients' passivity or dependence
- Personality disorder pathology compromising patients' ability to receive appropriate medical care

Much of the research on medical or somatic symptoms in patients with severe personality pathology comes from two highly productive groups: the McLean Study of Adult Development (a large prospective study of patients with BPD) and the team of a psychiatrist and family practitioner working together with other colleagues affiliated with the

Wright State School of Medicine and the Wright-Patterson Air Force Base [8–11]. The research by these teams underscores the bidirectional aspects of this topic: patients with personality disorders often have a variety of medical or somatic concerns, and patients with certain medical or somatic presentations sometimes have co-occurring personality disorder symptoms, often undiagnosed.

TFP principles can be useful to mental health providers treating those patients with PD diagnoses who present with associated physical symptoms and to medical specialists in varying roles and specialties who treat patients with PD symptoms. The critical TFP principles involved are (1) clarification of psychiatric diagnoses, including assessment of personality functioning, and medical diagnoses, when pertinent, (2) monitoring of the three channels of communication (what the patient says, how the patient behaves, and how the clinician feels), (3) the establishment and maintenance of a treatment frame, and (4) identification of dominant dyads and their role reversals within them. TFP principles are not magic, but they can help ground clinicians when faced with the specific chaos introduced by severe personality pathology. When medical or somatic complaints are part of this chaos, it automatically adds a dimension of trepidation and uncertainty for clinicians. Having a systematic, deliberate, and reliable approach to assessment and treatment addresses the countertransference experience of helplessness and impotence.

Mrs. G. Causes Difficulties for Her Primary Care Physician

Clinical vignette: Mrs. G., a widowed woman in her early 50s, estranged from her adult children, is referred by her primary care physician (PCP) to the psychiatric nurse practitioner in their group practice. The PCP had tried for over a year to manage Mrs. G.'s behaviors on his

(continued)

(continued)

own, but her consistent conflict with his office staff, her many phone calls and "emergency" pages, and her seemingly intractable headache complaints made this impossible, and he felt he needed help. The PCP had become aware of his chronic irritation with Mrs. G., given her demands for high doses of narcotics for her headaches, and the conflict among his office staff about management of her treatment. He feared setting any limits with Mrs. G. would increase her frustration, leading her to give him an "unfavorable" evaluation in the patient satisfaction rating program required by his accountable care organization.

Mrs. G. grudgingly agrees to meet with Mr. A., the psychiatric nurse practitioner. She describes to him a distant past of suicide attempts in her early 20s and her limited work history. She faults her children for their estrangement, blaming them for neglecting her after her husband died 5 years earlier. She is vague about her headache history, but waves away any suggestion that any intervention other than narcotics might be of use.

After his first meeting with Mrs. G., Mr. A. is comfortable conveying to her PCP a preliminary diagnostic impression. He describes her presentation as consistent with a patient who may have met criteria for BPD in the past, who now presents with some BPD traits but with primarily medical concerns. The PCP says he knows little about BPD patients and assumed they are all young and actively suicidal or self-injurious. Mr. A. reviews some key elements of effective management of patients with PD symptoms in general medicine practice. He describes (1) the process of making a PD diagnosis, (2) ongoing use of countertransference, (3) the utility of a treatment

(continued)

contract, and (4) identification of active dyads and their reversals.

Mrs. G.'s PCP welcomes the guidance from Mr. A. and starts by reviewing PD diagnostic criteria and sharing his impressions about Mrs. G. with his office staff. He considers his active countertransference reaction – irritation, fear, and impotence – and reflects on how changing his standard practice patterns with Mrs. G. might be harmful. At their next visit, Mrs. G.'s PCP describes a required frame for their treatment if they are to work together. This frame includes limits on the number of calls outside of work hours, a scheduled monthly meeting, and an expectation Mrs. G. would use available adjunctive non-narcotic interventions to help manage her headaches. Going forward, at times during their appointments when Mrs. G. would threaten or bully her PCP, he would recall Mr. A.'s description of dominant dyads in play and their reversals. Doing so allowed him to put into words Mrs. G.'s concerns (she would suffer alone, her doctor and his staff would be ineffective and uncaring) and describe the inverse he observed (Mrs. G. exerting control by threatening the doctor and his staff, the staff powerless and feeling compelled to accommodate her unreasonable requests). Over a number of months, Mrs. G.'s PCP begins to feel more in control; he is particularly relieved to have put in place a plan to limit the narcotics he prescribes.

Take Home Point: Medical professionals can use contracting to manage "difficult" patients even when they do not assume responsibility for these patients' psychiatric treatment.

7.3   In TFP Practice: The TFP Contract's Focus on Medical Sequelae of BPD and Other Potentially Treatment-Interfering Somatic Complaints

> - *The TFP contract will attempt to anticipate any medical concerns that may be treatment interfering.*
> - *The TFP contracting phase includes an expectation patients will cooperate with a medical evaluation of potentially treatment-interfering conditions.*
> - *The TFP contract addresses the possibility of medical complications related to self-injury (such as interference with wound healing).*
> - *The TFP therapist will refer back to (or renegotiate) the contract when somatic symptoms threaten the treatment.*

The TFP contract is designed with a specific goal: the establishment of a treatment frame guaranteeing the patient's consistent availability and participation and the safety of both the patient and therapist, allowing critical elements of the patient's object relations (or experience of self and others) to emerge in the transference. In the initial contracting phase, the therapist will actively explore any aspects of the patient's history that suggest ways medical or somatic concerns might undermine a patient's availability or participation. Some of these interfering medical concerns are common and described in the DSM-5 BPD diagnostic criteria: self-injury, binge eating, or consequences of physical fights, for example. Other medical or somatic concerns might not be specified in the standard nosology, but could similarly undermine treatment. Some examples might include the patient with chronic sleep difficulties, who might not be able to stay awake and alert during sessions, or the patient with a heightened sensitivity to medication side effects, who experiences unusual or extreme side effects with disruptions in functioning.

The TFP therapist may encounter a number of possible scenarios in the contracting phase related to physical or somatic symptoms. A common situation is the patient who maintains that a specific medical symptom such as fatigue or recurrent headaches would make commitment to the TFP frame impossible. The TFP therapist's approach would involve extensive questioning about the patient's history of medical evaluation and diagnosis, as well as ongoing compliance with recommendations made. The TFP therapist will use the contracting phase to obtain parallel information from other treaters involved to best clarify (1) the patient's medical diagnoses, (2) the recommendations made, and (3) the likelihood that the symptoms would, in fact, preclude compliance with the treatment frame. The TFP therapist will not go forward with treatment until these key questions are addressed. The therapist may be open to referring the patient to a more somatic symptom-focused treatment, such as cognitive-behavioral therapy, if during the contracting phase, management of chronic physical complaints emerges as a specific overriding concern.

A very different scenario is the patient presenting for treatment who *minimizes* the potential effects of an active medical issue. Consider the patient with an active anorexia nervosa seeking exploratory psychotherapy. The TFP therapist will bear in mind both the effects of this eating disorder's symptoms on the patient's ability to participate in treatment and the effects of the eating disorder symptoms on the therapist's level of anxiety. The patient with anorexia nervosa would be required by the TFP therapist to have a thorough medical evaluation with clearly established weight and electrolyte parameters in place before starting TFP treatment, if not a formal consultation with an eating disorder specialist. The goal of such parameters would be twofold: to insure the patient's cognitive capacity for the treatment and to reassure the therapist that concerning medical symptoms have been fully assessed and are actively monitored. Sometimes the TFP therapist will have to insist on this element of the contract, even as the patient protests that the medical concerns identified are not presently in evidence. This common quandary underscores again the utility of the treatment contracting process and the ways it can support the therapist during moments of confusion or self-doubt.

The BPD patient with active, recurrent, but not life-threatening, self-injury can present a particular problem, often coming to sessions with evidence of having engaged in self-injurious behavior. In this category are patients who come to session with evidence of having cut, scratched, or burnt themselves or engaged in head banging. In some cases, these patients will ask the therapist to inspect the site of injury. In other cases the patient may not mention new bruises, scarring, or even active bleeding, instead speaking about unrelated matters while leaving the therapist distracted and off balance. During the contracting phase, the TFP therapist may set limits on such behavior by establishing a requirement *in advance* that the patient first seek medical attention following any such episode before coming to psychotherapy. Such a requirement addresses the potential, albeit unspoken, provocation of coming to treatment with an evident but untreated wound; it also protects the clinician from being put in the uncomfortable position of passing judgment about the severity of a particular medical condition. (In this situation, the patient's behavior can reflect an expression of omnipotent control and a devaluing of the therapist – taking the therapist out of his or her role and therefore leaving the therapist uncomfortable, disarmed, and controlled. However, it may also reflect the patient's idealized experience of the treater as unusually caring or even omniscient and able to take care of problems magically.) In sum, contracting in advance about the involvement of primary care clinicians in the assessment of wounds associated with self-injury protects the therapist from having to operate in the state of concern and uncertainty typically engendered by the self-injurious patient.

In certain circumstances, a patient's medical or somatic concerns do not surface in the contracting phase. The TFP therapist will, when necessary, renegotiate the treatment contract with a patient when a particular medical or somatic complain comes to light and when this symptom risks undermining the treatment. Imagine the patient whose threats of suicide or self-injury resolve in the early months of treatment, but who then describes the new onset of sleep difficulties, which threaten engagement in studies and attendance and participation in treatment. The TFP therapist will be open to renegotiating the contract, conveying an expectation the patient would review this new symptom with a primary care clinician, follow standard sleep hygiene protocol, or even seek a sleep disorder evaluation, if indicated.

Ms. O. Comes to Her Psychotherapy Session with Self-Injury Wounds

Clinical vignette: Ms. O. trained as a nurse and worked in the cardiac ICU before persistent self-injury (head banging) and anxiety required she go on medical leave. Ms. O. was given diagnoses of social anxiety disorder, persistent depressive disorder, and unspecified personality disorder with borderline and dependent traits by her treatment team at the ambulatory center where she first received her psychiatric care.

After a year of outpatient treatment, Ms. O. had her first psychiatric hospitalization following a physical altercation with her younger sister, when it was revealed that her sister was dating a man Ms. O. had had a crush on during high school. The hospitalization resulted after emergency services were called because of Ms. O.'s bloodied knuckles, following her attempts to strike her sister, and the open wound on her forehead, after Ms. O. began banging her head following the fight. After this first hospitalization, Ms. O. ws reassigned to a team at a local intensive outpatient program (IOP) and given follow-up appointments in the general medical and neurology clinics.

During her first year of treatment before her hospitalization, Ms. O. often presented to her psychologist with a clearly visible wound, sometimes with breaks in the skin,

(continued)

(continued)

resulting from head-banging episodes. At the time of the transfer of Ms. O.'s care from this psychologist to the IOP, the psychologist confided to the psychiatrist and social worker at the program that she had frequently found the forehead wound distracting and disturbing. She recounted a number of episodes when Ms. O. would ask her to examine the wound, to weigh in on whether Ms. O. could go to work with the wound or instead whether she should go to the local urgent care center.

At the time of her intake at the IOP, Ms. O. met together with the psychiatrist who would be prescribing her medications and the social worker who would be her individual therapist. They reviewed with Ms. O. their diagnostic impression and described the respective responsibilities they would assume and they would expect from Ms. O. during her treatment. Ms. O. was surprised to learn she would have responsibilities in her treatment; she had considered herself "sick" and therefore expected her treaters to provide for her unconditionally, as her previous psychologist had. Ms. O. was even more surprised when her new team outlined their expectation that Ms. O. would be seen by a primary care clinician after any episode of self-injury; they explained that they would not meet with her until she had documentation of such a visit and medical clearance from a specialist (physician or nurse practitioner) who had examined her wound.

Ms. O. initially responded to this proposal with outrage and anger. She accused this new team of unnecessarily complicating her life, adding additional expense because of these proposed medical appointments, and displaying callousness about her psychiatric and medical conditions. The team tolerated her response but reiterated their terms, which Ms. O. eventually accepted.

Two months into her new treatment at the IOP, Ms. O. had a tense meeting with her supervisor at the ICU when

(continued)

negotiating an extension of her medical leave. She went home and punched the wall, injuring her wrist, and hit her head against the shower wall, reopening a healing wound. When she appeared at the IOP the next morning for her individual therapy session, she was instructed by her team to get a medical evaluation; she first protested, but did so reluctantly and returned for the IOP afternoon session. This episode marked the last time Ms. O. presented to treatment with a visible self-injury wound. Six months later, in one of her individual sessions, Ms. O. reflected on this pattern of behavior in past times: "I think I liked knowing I could get a certain kind of sympathy and attention by showing my injury; it felt good knowing I had some control. At the same time, and I'm embarrassed to say this, I liked watching my psychologist squirm a little bit. I know she didn't like blood but I could tell she didn't feel she could set a limit with me."

Take Home Point: Clinicians can use contracting to address a patient's provocative behavior, thus insuring the patient receives appropriate medical care and limiting disruption to the treatment.

7.4   The TFP Approach Aims to Minimize Iatrogenic Medical Complications

- *The TFP focus on clarification of diagnosis, including PD pathology, can assist clinicians in avoiding problematic and unnecessary interventions.*
- *The TFP approach can assist prescribers in limiting polypharmacy, often initiated during crises.*
- *The TFP approach can assist prescribers in confronting patient passivity about compromised self-care, sometimes associated with necessary medications (weight gain, elevated lipids).*

The medical consequences of undiagnosed or underdiagnosed personality disorder pathology can be serious and life-altering for patients. Research on BPD has confirmed the following: patients with BPD take a lot of different medications (including, but not limited to, psychotropics), often at high doses; the prevalence of BPD among the overweight and obese in mental health settings is significant; and a substantial number of patients with BPD have co-occurring substance use disorders, including opioid pain medication abuse or dependence [12–15]. TFP principles compel clinicians to consider many aspects of a patient's functioning; in doing so, the clinician will be prepared to consider both the standard DSM-5 personality disorder categories and the structural interview's more inclusive analysis of personality organization. How then would this approach help clinicians avoid iatrogenic complications including prescription of unnecessary or problematic medications?

Consider the clinician who does not actively consider the contribution of personality disorder pathology to the patient's presentation, instead conceptualizing the patient's PD symptoms (mood reactivity, rejection sensitivity, narcissistic injury) as exclusively reflecting a primary mood disorder diagnosis. This clinician can easily fall into a pattern of using multiple medications, often at high doses, in a fruitless attempt to address these symptoms. One critical consequence of such a pattern is exposing the patient to the various side effects of these medications. A number of the subtypes of psychiatric medications often prescribed to PD patients have serious, sometimes life-changing, medical side effects. This list includes:

- Antidepressant medications (weight gain, sexual side effects including diminished libido, sleep/wake cycle alteration, sedation, akathisia, elevated blood pressure)

(continued)

(continued)

- Atypical antipsychotic medications (weight gain, metabolic syndrome including elevated cholesterol and triglycerides, type II diabetes, akathisia, sedation)
- Mood stabilizers (weight gain, tremor, diabetes insipidus, life-threatening rash, sedation)
- Pain medications (opioid abuse or dependence)
- Attention deficit medications (stimulant abuse or dependence)

The systematic TFP approach of clarifying diagnosis is accompanied by a heightened sensitivity to the three channels of communication, including the treater's countertransference. The prescriber who makes a point of actively monitoring countertransference will question: Why am I prescribing so many medications to this patient? Why am I using medications at higher doses than I usually do? Why am I reluctant to recommend stopping a medication when it does not seem to be helping? Why am I accepting of a particular medication side effect with *this* patient, when I would ordinarily suggest changes in a medication regimen?

The clinician focused on countertransference reactions as part of prescribing may naturally gravitate toward a pattern of contracting with patients. Effective contracting is the cornerstone of a management approach aimed at minimizing iatrogenic complications. How would this work? The clinician aware of the specific dynamics arising when prescribing to patients with symptoms embedded in personality pathology will want to put in place in advance a defined process for decision-making about prescribing and active monitoring of medications prescribed. With many PD patients, this contracting process will include attention not only to compliance in taking the medications as directed but also attention to managing the effects of medications, including appropriate periodic testing or required behavior modification. Making use of evidence- or protocol-based regimens while targeting specifically identified symptoms, and making use of standardized rating scales to monitor response, can reduce the risk of countertransference-driven management. The prescribing of medication with PD patients may evoke the power of the internal representation of the "ideal object" in the patient's psychological functioning. Functioning with this wish for perfect care in the back of their minds, patients organized at a borderline level may reject any medication, even if helpful, that does not provide total relief. The clinician who is not attuned to this dynamic may fall into the trap of trying harder and harder to meet the patient's unrealistic expectations – hence, the polypharmacy, high doses of medications, and countertransference of frustration and impotence.

The focus on contracting can help the clinician limit polypharmacy, often begun when the patient is in crisis but then continued without further consideration even as the crisis resolves. The prescriber who is clear in advance about certain limits – "We will try this new medication for 1 month; if the symptom we are targeting persists after that time, we will begin a taper" – can avoid "surprising" the patient who may feel that a medication taper is depriving. Similarly, the prescriber who makes clear *in advance* the requirements for prescribing a particular agent will avoid an explosive confrontation going forward. The contract can include clear parameters for blood testing, active exercise, or monitoring of blood pressure.

Along with the focus on contracting, TFP principles guide the clinician to identify familiar patient-treater dyads, for example, the disempowered, vulnerable patient and the callous, oblivious treater. This dyad may contribute to countertransference pressures to *do something* for the patient – potentially leading clinicians to prescribe unusual combinations of medications, higher than customary doses, or supplies of medication unsafe in overdose. TFP's focus on the dyad and its reverse – in this case the empowered patient and the vulnerable prescriber concerned about side effects, medication misuse, or even overdose – can free the prescriber to think more clearly about medication management while being more comfortable setting limits with the patient and insuring self-protection.

Dr. A.'s "Treatment-Resistant Depression" Belies His Long-Standing Narcissistic Personality Pathology

Clinical vignette: Dr. A. is a psychologist in his mid-40s with long-standing moderate to severe borderline and narcissistic personality disorder symptoms. In his early 20s, Dr. A. displayed more frankly borderline symptoms with threats of self-injury and impulsive anger. Over time, Dr. A.'s symptoms reflected more prominent narcissistic traits, with striking grandiosity and exploitation of others. Throughout, Dr. A. conceptualized his difficulties as reflecting a "treatment-resistant major depression" leading him to many years of complex polypharmacy and supportive psychotherapy. Dr. A.'s psychotherapy supported his self-conception as someone vulnerable and easily mistreated by powerful, uncaring others, in his case his father and his sister, who financially supported Dr. A. for much of this period.

Dr. A. identified a prescribing psychiatrist, Dr. B., who considered himself an "expert psychopharmacologist" and who derived gratification from having a mental health professional like Dr. A. in his practice. This prescriber disdained personality disorder diagnoses, considering them stigmatizing and uniquely lacking in validity. Over the years Dr. A. tried many medication combinations, all with limited efficacy, but with significant side effects including weight gain, with a recently elevated hemoglobin A1C prediabetes screening test (from an atypical antipsychotic), and diminished libido and insomnia (from an MAOI antidepressant). Dr. A.'s delayed

(continued)

(continued)

sleep onset was highly disruptive, causing much concern to his wife, who often found herself getting up for work just as Dr. A. was going to sleep. She also felt chronically neglected because of their lack of sexual intimacy and less attracted to Dr. A. as he gained weight. Of note, Dr. A. came to expect increased financial support from his family to offset his partial employment, which he attributed to difficulty with his sleep/wake cycle.

Dr. A.'s relative stability was upended when his wife asked him for a separation. His despair and recurrence of suicidality led to his first psychiatric hospitalization. On admission to the inpatient unit, Dr. A.'s psychiatrist there, Dr. C., made a tentative diagnosis of a primary narcissistic personality disorder organized at a borderline level with prominent somatic concerns, some related to his medication regimen. Of particular concern were the abnormal findings on Dr. A.'s admission laboratory testing (including his lipid panel and fasting glucose level), his increasing abdominal girth, as well as his nightly need for multiple sleep aids to counter the effects of his antidepressant. Dr. C. was particularly alarmed when during his first phone contact with Dr. B., Dr. B. raised the possibility of adding a SSRI antidepressant to the MAOI – an unusual and possibly risky intervention Dr. B. assured Dr. C. he had tried before.

Dr. C. approached Dr. A. as he did all his inpatient cases, with an initial goal of generating a differential diagnosis. As noted, he began by conducting an extended evaluation, including exploration of aspects of personality functioning and level of organization. He identified Dr. A.'s personality disorder symptoms as primary, making the distinction between his long-standing alternating grandiosity and covert self-loathing, which at times looked like depressive affects, and actual sustained neurovegetative symptoms of major depression, which

(continued)

(continued)

were absent. Dr. C. also focused on Dr. A.'s list of physical and somatic concerns, including weight, sleep, and libido challenges, and their links to the medications he continued to take. Dr. C. first reviewed in detail with Dr. A. his tentative diagnostic impression, and they discussed what seemed accurate or misguided about this diagnostic impression. Dr. C. then presented to Dr. A. and his wife, father, and sister in a family meeting: his understanding of the central diagnostic issues; how he might suggest Dr. A. proceed after discharge, including a medication taper, not an increase in the number of medications and their associated risk; and appropriate psychotherapy options beyond supportive psychotherapy that might focus on (1) the psychological features underlying Dr. A.'s maladaptive personality functioning; (2) the roots of his reliance on "external" solutions, such as medication; and (3) the effects that his behavior and his toleration of medication have on others, including his wife.

Dr. A. received support from his wife, father, and sister to consider making a fundamental change in his treatment approach after many frustrating years. His family members outlined their long history of accepting his lack of progress in treatment and their more recent alarm at his emerging medical complications. They described their trepidation in confronting Dr. B., at the same time fearing that some of Dr. A.'s somatic symptoms might not be reversible unless there was a change in his treatment approach. The hospitalization served as a critical catalyst; despite some misgivings, Dr. A. was able to review his treatment, including the multiple somatic concerns he had come to accept as inevitable, and take steps to pursue treatment with a different approach.

Take Home Point: Distinguishing between a primary mood disorder and a primary or co-occurring personality disorder can be critical in identifying effective treatment interventions and minimizing iatrogenic complications.

7.5   TFP's Expectation for Change Will Dictate Exploration of Compromising Health-Related Lifestyle Choices

- *TFP will convey an expectation for change in the patient's life, including reduction of poor health-related lifestyle choices.*
- *The TFP contract will address compromising lifestyle choices when they present as treatment-interfering behaviors.*
- *The TFP therapist will be open to adding adjunctive treatments to assist patients in limiting compromising lifestyle choices.*

TFP as an individual psychotherapy modality emphasizes explicit clarification of the patient's personal goals and treatment goals. These goals serve as the "north star" of the treatment, orienting the therapist and patient and providing both with a way of assessing the efficacy of the treatment over time. TFP's focus on goals correlates with an understanding that many PD patients will be seeking some kind of character change, even if they are not able to articulate this aim as such. TFP goes beyond supportive interventions, with an expectation that patients' self-understanding and behavior and aspects of the patient's character will change over time.

TFP's focus on personal and treatment goals is closely tied to the therapist's expectation that for some patients, poor health-related lifestyle choices will emerge as critical topics, specifically as they interfere with achievement of these goals. These same poor health-related lifestyle choices can undermine the patient's full participation in treatment and/or the requirement for meaningful activity. Research has supported higher rates of the following among patients with BPD that does not remit [16]:

- Cigarette smoking
- Lack of regular exercise
- Daily use of sleeping medications
- Overuse use of pain medications
- Weekly alcohol use

In the contracting phase, TFP therapists will attend to any of these lifestyle choices that might undermine compliance with the treatment contract. The patient who is hung-over, or too sedated to actively participate in treatment, cannot meet the patient responsibilities defined in the treatment contract. As noted, the TFP therapist will also actively address ways these poor health-related lifestyle choices might interfere with a patient's stated personal and treatment goals. Take the patient with a significant pack-per-day pattern of cigarette use. The TFP therapist will actively address, along with the directly self-destructive impact of smoking, the discrepancy between the patient's goals (making new friends through a more active lifestyle) and a cigarette use habit that would make that less likely.

The TFP therapist will be open to introducing adjunctive treatments specifically created to address the poor health-related lifestyle choices listed. The individual psychotherapy can benefit from the patient's participation in a variety of programs with a focus on exercise, weight loss, ending smoking, limiting or stopping alcohol use, or improving sleep without medications. The TFP therapist would not expect the individual psychotherapy alone to address any or all of these maladaptive choices, but would instead convey openness to these other interventions.

Ms. M.'s Unhealthy Lifestyle Choices Undermine Her Treatment Goals

Clinical vignette: Ms. M., a 35-year-old divorced woman, working part-time, raising her son with little involvement by her former husband, presents to Dr. K. seeking treat-

(continued)

(continued)

ment. Ms. M. describes a history in her 20s of an extended individual psychotherapy that she found gratifying because of the support she received from her therapist at the time of her tumultuous divorce, but only somewhat helpful in addressing her primary difficulties: persistent loneliness and hopelessness about finding another romantic partner.

Ms. M. describes her extensive history with multiple prescribers trying a variety of psychiatric medications for what she describes as "major depression and panic attacks" with limited benefits and a variety of side effects, including weight gain of over 50 lbs., contributing to her current BMI of 30 (obese). At the time of her first meeting with Dr. K., she is no longer taking psychotropic medications, but makes little effort to lose the weight she had gained, a goal complicated by her one-and-a-half pack-per-day daily cigarette use, making exercise difficult. Ms. M. mentions that a number of eligible men in her community use a local health club, but she went only once after joining, feeling that the health club members looked down on her because of her smoking the one time she participated in a class there.

Dr. K. meets a number of times with Ms. M. with the purpose of completing his diagnostic assessment and clarifying Ms. M.'s current personal and treatment goals. Ms. M. is somewhat irritated by Dr. K.'s questions about treatment goals; she recounts her "desperation" at the time of her prior treatment and her expectation then that her therapist would "just be there for support" to help her navigate the turmoil of her separation and divorce. She blows up at Dr. K.: "You keep talking about goals and I don't understand your point! I saw a therapist because I needed someone on my side so that I could survive and take care of my son; that's what I need now, can't you understand that?"

(continued)

(continued)

Dr. K.'s initial diagnostic impression is that Ms. M. presents with a primary narcissistic disorder with a mix of obliviousness, fragility, and self-indulgence. Dr. K. notes that Ms. M.'s narcissistic fragility makes it difficult for her to convey directly her desire to begin dating with a goal of identifying a partner. At the same time, Dr. K. suspects Ms. M. has limited insight into the impact her behaviors have on others, including her cigarette smoking. When he raises this issue tentatively, Ms. M. waves away his concern: "In Europe everyone smokes; they don't have the hang-ups people have in this country."

Dr. K. has an opportunity to speak with Ms. M.'s prior therapist. This conversation confirms Dr. K.'s suspicion that their treatment was limited by the implicit threat of Ms. M.'s anger. He learns that the prior therapist felt that Ms. M. would only accept one specific version of her multiple challenges, i.e., that she was a sensitive, trusting "doormat," getting the short end of the stick from more aggressive, self-serving others.

In the contracting phase, Dr. K. is frank with Ms. M. about the likely impact of choices she makes (smoking, lack of exercise) on her goals. Ms. M. is clearly annoyed with Dr. K. for sharing this observation. Dr. K. considers their discussion as part of the contracting process to be a helpful window into the likely trajectory of the treatment and exploration of the dominant dyad ("chump" being mistreated by selfish others) and its inverse (in this case, controlling figure expecting others to accommodate her without questioning).

Despite her misgivings, Ms. M. agrees to move forward with treatment as outlined in her contract with Dr. K. Ms. M.'s protests about Dr. K.'s focus on certain of her lifestyle choices diminish over time. Ms. M. decides on her own first to access behavioral treatment for her

(continued)

(continued)

smoking and then to join a weight reduction group in her community. Dr. K. consistently links Ms. M.'s lifestyle choices to her stated treatment goals; eventually Ms. M. stops ascribing critical judgment about her choices to Dr. M. and focuses more on her own ambivalence about self-care.

Take Home Point: The therapist should actively address poor lifestyle choices when such choices clearly interfere with personal goals identified during the assessment and contracting phase.

7.6   TFP's Approach Aims to Limit Medical Disability as an Expression of PD Pathology

- *Medical or somatic symptoms are associated with disability status for certain patients with BPD and other PD presentations.*
- *The TFP attendance and work or study requirements implicitly address passivity or parasitism, sometimes expressed as medical or somatic symptoms.*
- *Claims of medical disability can be difficult to contest or verify; clinicians may be stymied when confronting medical complaints that reflect a factitious disorder or malingering.*

Multiple studies have identified a clear link between the diagnosis of BPD and both psychiatric and medical disability status. Researchers have examined this phenomenon from different perspectives: BPD patients diagnosed during hospitalization, random patients presenting for disability screened for PD symptoms, follow-up of patients presenting for work-related physical disability claims, and patients screened in an internal medicine clinic using BPD self-report measures [17–20]. One researcher has concluded that for some BPD patients, "[medical disability] compensation provides societal verification of somatic dysfunction" [1].

As noted, TFP requires a patient to engage in meaningful volunteer or paid work or studies. If a patient is assessed as incapable of this kind of engagement in life, they are referred to a therapy that has a goal of maintaining stability rather than one of increasing autonomous functioning. This require-ment directly confronts a common and concerning trajectory for many BPD patients: a path from symptomatic patient to one with disability status who has given up on life goals. Sometimes the disability is psychiatric, and other times the disability is medical. (This phenomenon is further complicated by the trajectory sometimes observed that certain BPD patients "migrate" from primarily psychiatric to primarily medical presentations when psychiatric benefits are restricted.) A path returning from disability to employment is a notori-ously challenging one, achievable but at significant odds [21].

The TFP therapist introduces the work or study expecta-tion in the earliest stages of contracting. The therapist does not "wait and see," nor does the therapist qualify the require-ment for individual patients, if TFP is to be the treatment offered. Of course, the TFP therapist may conclude a patient requires a different kind of approach. However, in some cases when TFP may be the appropriate treatment, medical or somatic concerns pose obstacles in the contracting phase by precluding the patient from making the commitment to the treatment frame or to the work or study obligation. The TFP therapist will ask: Has the patient had the physical symptoms evaluated? What is the working medical diagnosis? Has the patient been given instructions about how to manage this symptom? If so, has the patient followed these instructions?

A subset of patients with moderate to severe personality disorder pathology will come to rely on family or government financial support either through passivity or more active exploitation or parasitism. This particular pattern of behavior often co-occurs with the development of medical or somatic symptoms. In such a case, the patient will expect financial support because of a medical or somatic complaint, sometimes with endorsement of medical specialists involved, but sometimes without. The therapist who is offering a treatment with a goal of significant life change will have to address the subject of these somatic or medical concerns head-on. This will involve communication with medical treaters and pointed questioning about the feasibility of full attendance and meaningful daily activity. Often the therapist is left to interpret for the patient conflicting motives: one, to make significant changes with a move toward autonomy, and another, to be cared for by an unquestioning and undemanding source of support.

The TFP therapist may have to question whether the TFP modality is appropriate for certain patients presenting with physical or somatic concerns. Why should that be? The emergence of physical symptoms as a limitation for either attendance or participation in treatment or compliance with the work or study requirement automatically brings into the treatment the third party of medical provider. In this case the therapist may find himself on one side of a "split" not easily bridged. In many cases, the therapist may have to defer to the expertise of the medical specialist. Sometimes this medical expertise reflects a straightforward exchange of information; other times involvement of the third-party medical expert reflects the patient's partially or fully unconscious motivation to retaliate for the anger and humiliation resulting from the introduction of increased commitments. The therapist in this situation will be facing a patient's more aggressive, even destructive side, which could be communicated through a medical expert who does not have an appreciation of the role of personality disorder pathology.

The literature on the limits of treatability of certain PD patients stresses the continuum from more severe borderline or narcissistic pathology, through "malignant narcissism" notable for ego-syntonic aggression and circumscribed antisocial traits, to frank antisocial personality disorder [22]. A patient's medical or somatic concerns can be closely linked to this discussion of treatability. Why should this be so? Consideration of treatability is linked to the issue of "secondary gain of illness" or conscious or unconscious "benefits" a patient derives from assuming the role of patient. The TFP therapist may feel confident directly addressing the issue of "secondary gain" when a patient's symptoms are primarily behavioral. When the symptoms associated with secondary gain are partially or exclusively medical, as noted, the TFP therapist is required to work with medical specialists. The questions follow naturally: Is the patient physically capable of attending treatment? Is the patient physically able to work or participate in studies? Who makes this decision? Is the conclusion about this capability a dynamic or static one? Who makes the decision about application for medical disability, either through private insurance or a government program?

Clinicians are understandably concerned about minimizing or contesting a patient's complaints of physical discomfort. On the other hand, it is reasonable to expect that physical symptoms will have psychological significance for patients with PD symptoms. The TFP therapist remains sensitive to the meaning of medical and somatic symptoms as they emerge in the treatment. This sensitivity is not expressed in a caricatured, orthodox psychoanalytic way (authoritatively interpreting all physical symptoms as psychodynamically significant), but with an acceptance of a certain ambiguity that must be better understood. That said, the patient resolutely closed to exploration of the meaning of somatic symptoms should prompt the therapist to consider the limits of treatability with the TFP model.

> *Mr. O.'s Personality Disorder-Related Decline in Functioning Leads Ineffably to His Application for Medical Disability*
>
> *Clinical vignette: After quitting his first job after college, Mr. O moves into his parents' basement. He tells his parents the 1 year of a "nine-to-five grind" of an office*

(continued)

(continued)

job was intolerable and describes his plan to develop his skills playing the guitar and writing songs. For 6 months, Mr. O. spends most of his time watching television and smoking marijuana and occasionally seeing friends at a local bar, but otherwise isolating himself. Mr. O. becomes indignant when his parents suggest he look for work, assuring them he is working on his "craft" that he antici-pates will allow him to earn money sometime in the future.

Mr. O. develops a pattern of staying up all night and sleeping much of the day. He complies with his parents' requirement that he meet with a psychiatrist, who diagno-ses Mr. O. with a primary sleep disorder and prescribes a series of sedative-hypnotic medications that Mr. O. takes inconsistently. A brief trial of cognitive-behavioral ther-apy (CBT) for insomnia is aborted after Mr. O. misses three sessions in a row. Mr. O. is then started on an anti-depressant medication although he denies any depression symptoms other than disturbed sleep; he is unable to tol-erate the medication and stops it on his own after 2 weeks. When his parents give Mr. O. an ultimatum that he either look for work or move out, Mr. O. protests that they are victimizing him by blaming him for his disabling sleep disorder. Mr. O.'s psychiatrist then refers him to a sleep disorder specialist who recommends a sleep study, which has equivocal results. After another 6 months, Mr. O. tells his parents he may need to seek help from a nationally known sleep disorder specialist out of state because of his intractable symptoms. He also mentions that he is consid-ering filing papers for medical disability.

Mr. O.'s parents then insist he see a psychologist for a second opinion. Dr. P. meets three times with Mr. O. and once with Mr. O. and his parents. Dr. P. speaks with Mr. O.'s psychiatrist, cognitive-behavioral therapist, and sleep disorder specialist. Dr. P. meets with Mr. O. and his parents and outlines his thinking, including his diagnos-tic considerations and requirements for treatment.

(continued)

Mr. O. and his parents are surprised when Dr. P. emphasizes Mr. O.'s long-standing maladaptive coping mechanisms and describes personality disorder symptoms, a term unfamiliar to them. They wonder why Dr. P. is not prioritizing either the sleep disorder (Mr. O.'s focus) or a possible depression (his parents' concern). Dr. O. outlines a set of requirements for treatment for both Mr. O. and his parents. These include expectations that (1) Mr. O. will follow the recommendations of clinicians involved, including compliance with medication as written and CBT for insomnia, (2) Mr. O. will commit to meaningful work or studies as part of his treatment with Dr. P., and (3) Mr. O.'s parents will themselves seek help for setting a limit on their support should Mr. O. fail to comply with his obligations. Only Dr. P.'s firm instructions and the ongoing support of a family therapist are enough to help Mr. O.'s parents stay resolute in their requirements and thus help Mr. O. avoid drifting toward medical disability.

Take Home Point: Personality disorder pathology can be closely associated with medical or psychiatric disability, requiring clinicians to proactively address such a possibility with clear but firm expectations.

7.7   TFP Principles for Clinicians Providing Medical Care for Patients with PD Symptoms

- *Patients with PD pathology can pose multiple, unusual challenges to medical professionals, presenting with psychiatric or medical complaints or both.*
- *Medical professionals will have varying levels of familiarity with PD pathology; some may make a PD*

(continued)

(continued)

diagnosis, and others will employ strategies designed for treating "the difficult patient."
- *Medical professionals can use TFP principles when treating patients with PD symptoms without assuming responsibility for their psychiatric care.*
- *TFP principles can benefit medical professionals treating patients with subsyndromal PD presentations, sometimes evidenced by compromised compliance.*

Studies suggest that clinicians in primary care medical settings likely treat a significant number of patients with BPD. One study using structured interviews in an urban outpatient primary care setting found a prevalence rate of 6.4 %; a second study using self-report measures found rates of borderline symptomatology in a resident-provider primary care clinic of approximately 25% [23, 24]. These rates are notably higher than those in community samples (estimated to be approximately 2 %) but lower than some estimates in mental health settings (15–50 %) [25, 26]. Such figures are for BPD only; rates including other personality disorder pathology and subsyndromal personality disorder presentations would, of course, be much higher.

These statistics are reflected in the various clinical situations medical professionals encounter in their practices. Sansone and Sansone outlined familiar manifestations of underlying BPD pathology encountered in medical settings. These different permutations include:

1. PD patients presenting to medical professionals with primarily psychiatric complaints
2. Patients presenting to medical professionals with medical complaints directly related to their PD disorder
3. Patients with PD diagnoses whose access to general medical care is somehow compromised by a habitual maladap-

tive experience of others (in this case medical professionals or office staff).

The categories outlined above suggest relatively discrete patterns of presentation when, in fact, clinical experience suggests PD patients over time can present with a mix of the patterns described.

The patients described in category 1 are those who bring complaints related directly to psychiatric symptoms to their medical providers. As noted, some of these complaints are clearly the result of PD symptoms, as with self-injury or overdoses (recovery from self-injury may be complicated in some cases when BPD patients engage in medically self-sabotaging behavior) [27]. PD patients may first encounter primary care or specialist providers when seeking treatment for substance use or eating disorders or conditions directly related to impulsivity such as sequelae to unsafe sex or reckless driving. In addition, primary care clinicians may be the first to prescribe medications for patients describing the particular dysphoria of BPD, often reflecting mood reactivity or boredom and emptiness, easily mistaken for a primary depressive disorder. Medical professionals will also see PD patients who present for treatment related to other commonly co-occurring psychiatric conditions, often related to self-regulation, including anxiety, attention, or sleep disorders.

The patients falling into category 2, those with a primary medical complaint, may be the most confusing to medical professionals treating them. Investigators have examined the association between BPD and a number of medical disorders and found varying results. Some possible scenarios faced by clinicians include (1) the patient with medical complaints observed to have frequent co-occurrence with PD presentations, (2) the patient with medical complaints that may be related to common psychiatric treatments for PD symptoms, or (3) the patient who happens to have a personality disorder presenting for routine care, whose medical complaints are independent of PD symptoms.

Some common medical presentations seen to different degrees in PD patients include:

- Migraine headaches
- Chronic fatigue syndrome
- Multiple chemical sensitivities
- Temporomandibular disorders
- Sleep disorders and need for standing sleep medications
- Poor health-related lifestyle choices
- Obesity with associated hypertension, diabetes, osteoarthritis, or urinary incontinence
- Chronic pain symptoms
- Chronic opioid use for pain management
- Irritable bowel syndrome
- Fibromyalgia

As outlined earlier, some of these medical complaints have been noted to have higher than expected co-occurrence rates among patients with BPD (e.g., chronic pain, fibromyalgia, and obesity) [28–30]. Others may either be iatrogenically induced or additionally complicated by certain routine psychiatric interventions (obesity, chronic opioid use for pain, and standing sleep medications). Still other medical symptoms may reflect Somatic Symptom Disorder or related conditions, given the link supported by multiple studies between BPD and somatic preoccupation of different kinds [31, 32].

Consider category 3, the patient who does not identify specific psychiatric concerns or medical concerns but nevertheless causes disruption for medical practitioners [33]. Because this patient does not necessarily identify himself or herself as a psychiatric patient, the medical professional may not automatically link disruptive behavior to a personality disorder diagnosis. Similarly, while as noted certain medical conditions are closely associated with co-occurring PD diagnoses, it is reasonable to expect that some PD patients will have other medical conditions or complaints that do not necessarily alert the treater to a possible concurrent PD presentation.

The PD patient without explicit medical or psychiatric complaints may earn a reputation as "the difficult patient." This patient may be one who is persistently non-compliant, doesn't come for needed appointments, or comes *too* frequently, without clear needs. Research confirms that a subset of BPD patients, for example, are unusually high utilizers of primary care and medical specialist services [34]. Often the difficult patient generates an excessive number of phone calls or agitates for multiple prescriptions of different kinds, causing the medical professional to feel compelled to set limits. One study of BPD patients in primary care settings identified patterns of disruptive behavior in the medical setting, including yelling, screaming, verbal threatening, refusing to talk with medical staff, and talking badly about medical staff to family and friends (this study did not find a link between BPD and physical violence in medical settings) [31].

Sansone and Sansone outlined the following clinical situations in medical practice that would suggest the need for consideration of PD pathology:

- Splitting among office staff (i.e., unusual disagreements about management related to a specific patient)
- Chronic difficulties with self-regulation
- Self-harm including medical self-sabotage
- Rapid development of intense transferences, positive and negative, to staff members
- Premature familiarity with clinicians and staff
- Response to limit setting with regressed or childlike behavior
- Testing of professional boundaries
- Testing of caring by way of unusual requests for services
- Unusual or polysymptomatic presentations
- Histories of multiple prior treaters

A TFP-informed approach for medical professionals should be, by necessity, succinct and direct. In many, if not most, situations, medical professionals will not have the time to engage a patient in an extended evaluation of behavioral symptoms. The TFP approach would be guided by an appreciation of countertransference reactions: In this treatment relationship, how does the clinician feel? Common countertransference reactions for medical professionals treating patients with severe PD symptoms can include irritation, hate, or avoidance, often reflecting an experience of feeling devalued, deskilled, or even endangered. Alternatively, medical professionals can sometimes feel an unusual identification, protectiveness, or atypical closeness when treating PD patients.

The clinician prompted by an unusual countertransference reaction will consider the possibility of a PD diagnosis. This process doesn't necessarily have to involve the patient filling out questionnaires or walking through a diagnostic algorithm with the patient – it is more a personal clinical impression. Along with consideration of a PD diagnosis, the clinician will begin to consider the dominant object relations, or dyads, in play, representations of self and others that reflect the patient's internal object world. Often these dyads begin with the patient feeling aggrieved in some way, describing himself or herself as deprived or victimized, for example. This can "flip": the nurse feels she is suffering (from complaints, phone calls, angry outbursts) from a callous and victimizing *patient*. Another possibility is the well-cared-for patient gratified by the always available and limitlessly generous physician. This may work for a while until something interferes with the maintenance of this dyad; the physician may then witness a rapid shift from the patient's highly idealizing to a powerfully devaluing experience of the clinician.

The process of "naming the actors" or putting into words the clinician's appreciation of the dominant object relations can be useful. Here are some scenarios:

- A patient seeing himself as deprived and his nurse practitioner as withholding, engaging multiple other clinicians because of his dissatisfaction
- A controlling, omnipotent patient "bossing around" a cowed physician's assistant by coming late to appointments and demanding prescriptions
- A patient who sees herself as dependent and gratified clinging to her nurse as if he is a perfect provider, hanging around the office and leaving the nurse gifts and cards

The process of "naming the actors" or identifying the dominant object relations can be containing, conveying to the patient that the medical professional has an understanding of his or her experience. More importantly, naming the actors "puts on the table" something that may have been unspoken or acted out, giving the clinician an opportunity to look with the patient at what is happening in their relationship. Identification of the dominant object relations is coupled with an awareness of a possible reversal in the dyad: as noted above, the patient who feels poorly treated and controlled can quickly become the patient who causes disruption in the office because of how he treats the staff or controls the clinicians.

The clinician linking an unusual countertransference reaction with any of the clinical situations listed above (in the Sansone and Sansone chart) will also be prompted to attend to the treatment frame – i.e., the basic elements of patient engagement and cooperation necessary for the clinician to provide care in a safe and reasonable manner. Medical and surgical clinicians may be moved to focus on the treatment frame when ad hoc interventions with the PD patient are unsuccessful. It may be common for the clinician to try to "reason" with the patient, ending in failure; another reflexive but ill-advised approach is to respond to the patient with in-kind aggression, as in "Don't talk to me like that!" or "Control yourself and settle down!" The treatment frame and its associated stability help to address elements of PD pathology reflected in the list of concerning behaviors seen in medical settings. These elements include variable reality testing and transient paranoia; rejection sensitivity, neediness, impulsivity, and "affect storms"; and identity diffusion and associated fragmentation.

What is the point of the contract for the medical professional? Imagine the clinician with a growing awareness of an unusual countertransference reaction such as loathing or vulnerability *or* unusual closeness or a motivation to "rescue" a patient. The contract helps anchor the treatment and gives the clinician a way to communicate: "We need these parameters in place so that I can think clearly and provide you with good care." The contract isn't the same as office rules; the contract is a mutually agreed-upon set of obligations for both parties. The medical professional monitoring her countertransference, identifying the dominant object relations dyads in play, and proactive in establishing a treatment contract with a "difficult" patient will nevertheless expect the contract to be challenged. The clinician explains the rationale for the contract: "I can't give you the care you deserve when you come late, yell at the office staff, and demand prescriptions without question. Here is a plan with responsibilities defined for both of us." The clinician also expects to revisit the contract with the patient: "You're anxious today about your pain medications and you're raising your voice. We have an agreement that allows me to take care of you to the best of my abilities. When you yell at me that's not possible."

The utility of contracting with patients extends from those patients with clear personality disorder pathology to those with subsyndromal presentations and to patients who, for whatever reason, have challenges with compliance. Research has underscored the clinical significance of the subsyndromal PD presentation; in fact, the presence of just *one* BPD feature has been shown to have an impact on key indices of functioning [35]. Emerging data supports a hypothesis that PD symptoms generally, and BPD symptoms in particular, are associated with both increased chronic health problems *and* impairment in functioning (pain, fatigue, negative perceptions of overall health), *independent of the presence of chronic health problems* [36]. Taken together, these observations suggest that patients who may not meet DSM-5 PD criteria, who may have as few as one PD symptom, could nevertheless have behaviors leading to compromised medical care. The medical professional engaged with a patient without a clear PD diagnosis, but with challenges to compliance, can use contracting in this context as well. The physician or nurse who establishes expectations in advance and has a clear agreement as a point of reference during the course of treatment can avoid expectable frustration and lost time.

Mr. O.'s Non-compliance Leads His Nurse Practitioner to Seek Consultation

Clinical vignette: Mr. R., a nurse practitioner, dreaded the days he saw Mr. O.'s name on his schedule. Mr. O. was a single man in his late 20s who first presented to Mr. R.'s clinic for routine medical care. Mr. R. learned that Mr. O. had been diagnosed with attention deficit disorder as a child and depression in his early 20s, but now avoided all psychiatric care because of negative experiences with what Mr. O. called "useless shrinks."

Mr. O. began to complain to Mr. R. about sleep problems. Mr. R. proceeded in his standard way, first reviewing possible contributing factors to this new problem and then describing standard sleep hygiene interventions. Mr. O. quickly became impatient with Mr. R., insisting on medication for his insomnia, intimating it would be Mr. R.'s fault if Mr. O. were to lose his job because of his sleep problems. Mr. R. was aware of feeling a mix of irritation and fear, concerned he might be depriving Mr. O. of symptom relief and pressured to prescribe medications despite his reservations. Over the course of months, Mr. R. prescribed a number of medications – sedative-hypnotics, anxiolytics, sedating antidepressants, and atypical antipsychotics – none of which helped Mr. O. for very long.

(continued)

(continued)

Mr. R.'s frustrations grew as Mr. O. often missed appointments, called insisting prescriptions be sent to him between visits, sometimes reporting losing prescriptions, often asking for medication at higher than recommended doses, and then protesting if Mr. R. expressed concerns. Mr. O. often made oblique references to his desperation related to his insomnia, which made Mr. R. even more anxious, given that the medications he had prescribed were possibly toxic in overdose. Mr. R. had had experience with patients with substance use disorders wanting medications from him, but he noted Mr. O. would agitate just as aggressively for medications like sedating antidepressants or atypical antipsychotic as those more commonly abused like benzodiazepines.

Mr. R.'s growing anxiety led him to seek out consultation with Ms. E., the social worker at his clinic. Ms. E. encouraged Mr. R. to begin by reconsidering Mr. O.'s diagnoses; she suggested that along with possible mood, attention, and sleep disorder symptoms, Mr. R.'s experience of Mr. O. suggested the possible contribution of personality disorder symptoms. Ms. E. strongly emphasized Mr. R.'s exploration of his countertransference with Mr. O., specifically his sense of impotence and fear despite Mr. O.'s accusations that Mr. R. was, at times, uncaring and ineffectual. Ms. E. suggested Mr. R.'s countertransference was a common one for clinicians treating patients with certain personality traits, marked by the patient's ability to exert a powerful control, despite the clinician's best intentions.

Ms. E. introduced to Mr. R. the idea of negotiating with Mr. O. a contract required for their continued treatment relationship. She suggested Mr. R. schedule extra time to do this, to avoid a rushed, frantic appointment often caused by Mr. O.'s tardiness. Mr. O. was only marginally

(continued)

(continued)

cooperative with negotiation of a treatment contract, but Mr. R. held fast and repeatedly brought Mr. O.'s attention to their respective responsibilities in the treatment. Mr. R. reviewed issues like lateness, missed appointments, and overuse of medication. Ms. E. had warned Mr. R. that Mr. O. would likely challenge the terms of the contract, which he did, but having the contract in place greatly reduced Mr. R.'s sense of assault and resignation, allowing him to think more clearly than had been possible before.

Take Home Point: Medical professionals can use the contracting process to address common challenges encountered when treating patients with significant personality disorder pathology in general medical settings.

References

1. Sansone R, Sansone L. Borderline personality disorder in the medical setting: unmasking and managing the difficult patient. New York: Nova Science Publishers, Inc; 2007.
2. Gunderson JG, Links PS. Borderline personality disorder: a clinical guide. 2nd ed. Arlington, VA: American Psychiatric Publishing; 2008.
3. Sansone RA, Sansone LA, Wiederman MW. Borderline personality disorder and health care utilization in a primary care setting. South Med J. 1996;89:1162–5.
4. Morgan TA, Zimmerman M. Is borderline personality disorder underdiagnosed and bipolar disorder overdiagnosed? In: Choi-Kain LW, Gunderson JG, editors. Borderline personality and mood disorders: comorbidity and controversy. New York: Springer; 2015. p. 65–78.
5. Dubovsky AN, Kiefer MM. Borderline personality disorder in the primary care setting. Med Clin. 2014;98(5):1049–64.

6. Ricke AK, Lee MJ, Chambers JE. The difficult patient: border-line personality disorder in the obstetrics and gynecological patient. Obstet Gynecol Surv. 2012;67(8):495–502.

7. Zerbo E, Cohen S, Bielska W, Caligor E. Transference-focused psychotherapy in the general psychiatry residency: a useful and applicable model for residents in acute clinical settings. Psychodyn Psychiatry. 2013;41(1):163–81.

8. Frankenberg FR, Zanarini MC. The association between border-line personality disorder and chronic medical illnesses, poor health-related lifestyle choices, and costly forms of health care utilization. J Clin Psychiatry. 2004;65:1660–5.

9. Frankenberg FR, Zanarini MC. Relationship between cumula-tive BMI and symptomatic, psychosocial, and medical outcomes in patients with borderline personality disorder. J Pers Disord. 2011;25:421–31.

10. Sansone RA, Wiederman MW, Sansone LA. The relationship between borderline personality symptomatology and health care utilization among women in an HMO setting. Am J Manag Care. 1996;2:515–8.

11. Sansone RA, Sansone LA. Borderline personality disorder: the enigma. Prim Care Rep. 2000;6:219–26.

12. Sansone RA, Rytwinski D, Gaither GA. Borderline personality and psychotropic medication prescription in an outpatient psy-chiatry clinic. Compr Psychiatry. 2003;44:454–8.

13. Makela EH, Moeller KE, Fullen JE, Gunel E. Medication utili-zation patterns and methods of suicidality in borderline person-ality disorder. Ann Pharmacother. 2006;40:49–52.

14. Sansone RA, Sansone LA, Morris DW. Prevalence of borderline personality symptoms in two groups of obese subjects. Am J Psychiatry. 1996;153:117–8.

15. Sansone RA, Whitecar P, Meier BP, Murry A. The prevalence of borderline personality among primary care patients with chronic pain. Gen Hosp Psychiatry. 2001;23:193–7.

16. Keuroghliam AS, Frankenberg FR, Zanarini MC. The relation-ship of chronic medical illnesses, poor health-related lifestyle choices, and health care utilization to recovery status in border-line patients over a decade of prospective follow-up. J Psychiatr Res. 2013;47:1499–506.

17. Zanarini MC, Jacoby RJ, Frankenberg FR, Reich DB, Fitzmaurice G. The 10-year course of social security disability income reported by patients with borderline personality disorder and axis II comparison subjects. J Pers Disord. 2009;23(4):346–56.

18. Mikkelsen EJ. The psychology of disability. Psychiatr Ann. 1977;7:90–9.
19. Burton K, Polatin PB, Gatchel RJ. Psychosocial factors and the rehabilitation of patients with chronic work-related upper extremity disorders. J Occup Rehabil. 1997;7:139–53.
20. Sansone RA, Butler M, Dakroub H, Pole M. Borderline personality symptomatology and employment disability among outpatients in an internal medicine clinic. Primary Care Companion. 2006;8:153–7.
21. Stone M. The fate of borderline patients: successful outcome and psychiatric practice. New York: Guilford Press; 1990.
22. Kernberg OK. The almost untreatable narcissistic patient. J Am Psychoanal Assoc. 2007;55(2):503–39.
23. Gross R, Olfson M, Gameroff M, Shea S, et al. Borderline personality disorder in primary care. Arch Int Med. 2002;162:53–60.
24. Sansone RA, Weiderman M, Sansone LA. Medically self-harming behavior and its relationship to borderline personality symptoms and somatic preoccupation among internal medicine patients. J Nerv Ment Dis. 2000;188:45–7.
25. Grant BF, Chou SP, Goldstein RB, Huang B, Stinson FS, Saha TD, et al. Prevalence, correlates, disability, and comorbidity of DSM-IV borderline personality disorder: results from the wave 2 national epidemiologic survey on alcohol and related conditions. J Clin Psychiatry. 2008;69(4):533–45.
26. Widiger TA, Weissman MM. Epidemiology or borderline personality disorder. Hosp Community Psychiatry. 1991;42(10):1015–21.
27. Sansone RA, Wiederman M, Sansone LA, Mehnert-Kay S. Sabotaging one's own medical care. Arch Fam Med. 1997;6:583–6.
28. Sansone RA, Sansone LA. Chronic pain syndromes and borderline personality. Innove Clin Neurosci. 2012;9(1):10–4.
29. Sansone RA, Hawkins R. Fibromyalgia, borderline personality, and opioid prescription. Gen Hosp Psychiatry. 2004;26:415–6.
30. Sansone RA, Wiederman MW, Monteith D. Obesity, borderline personality symptomatology, and body image among women in a psychiatric outpatient setting. Int J Eat Disord. 2001;29:76–9.
31. Sansone RA, Weiderman MW, Sansone LA. Adult somatic preoccupation and its relationship to childhood trauma. Violence Vict. 2001;16:39–48.
32. Hudziak JJ, Boffeli TJ, Kriesman JJ, Battaglia MM. Clinical study of the relation of borderline personality disorder to Briquet's

syndrome (hysteria), somatization disorder, antisocial personality disorder, and substance abuse disorder. Am J Psychiatry. 1996;153:1598–606.

33. Sansone RA, Gentille J, Markert RJ. Drug allergies among patients with borderline personality symptomatology. Gen Hosp Psychiatry. 2000;22:289–90.

34. Sansone RA, Weiderman MW, Sansone LA. Borderline personality symptomatology, experience of multiple types of trauma, and health care utilization among women in a primary care setting. J Clin Psychiatry. 1998;59:108–11.

35. Zimmerman M, Chelminski I, Young D, Dalyrmple K, Martinez J. Does the presence of one feature of borderline personality disorder have clinical significance? Implications for dimensional ratings of personality disorders. J Clin Psychiatry. 2012;73(1):8–12.

36. Powers AD, Oltmanns TF. Personality disorders and physical health: a longitudinal examination of physical functioning, healthcare utilization, and health-related behaviors in middle-aged adults. J Pers Disord. 2012;26(4):524–38.

Chapter 8
Transference-Focused Psychotherapy (TFP) Principles in Psychiatry Residency Training

1. *TFP's unified theory offers psychiatry residents an organizing and practical psychodynamically-informed approach to conceptualizing a patient's clinical presentation and providing patient care.*
2. *TFP offers psychiatry residents a clearly described way to use psychodynamic principles in multiple clinical situations beyond the individual psychotherapy setting.*
3. *TFP training offers psychiatry residents an accessible, coherent approach to the practice of individual psychodynamic psychotherapy.*
4. *TFP training offers psychiatry residents a model for understanding personality pathology and the behavior of PD patients in a variety of settings, helping to fill the gap in many residency programs' education about personality disorders.*
5. *The structural interview's deliberate integration of roles of physician, psychiatrist, and psychodynamic psychotherapist fits well with the responsibilities of psychiatry trainees.*
6. *TFP training can assist psychiatry trainees in their introduction to risk management concerns.*

© Springer International Publishing Switzerland 2016   231
R.G. Hersh et al., *Fundamentals of Transference-Focused Psychotherapy*, DOI 10.1007/978-3-319-44091-0_8

8.1   Introduction

Transference-focused psychotherapy (TFP) and its theories and approach to patient care have only recently been introduced into psychiatry residency training education in limited pilot programs [1, 2]. These pilot programs have underscored the potential utility of exposing psychiatry trainees to the theory and practice of TFP with two goals: first, to provide an overarching psychodynamic approach to understanding patients and organizing their treatment in the variety of settings where residents see patients and, second, to offer a succinct and organizing model for conducting individual psychotherapy meeting the Accreditation Council for Graduate Medical Education (ACGME) requirement for residents' exposure to psychodynamic psychotherapy practice. Experience with these pilot programs for TFP training during residency suggests that it may be useful to think of TFP as (1) a set of psychodynamically informed tools for residents to use in the many acute care settings where they see patients during training *and* (2) a template for the practice of individual psychotherapy for a variety of patients, useful beyond the more narrow category of those with borderline personality disorder (BPD), the patient population that has been the focus of TFP research.

Psychiatry residents begin their training with a focus on a "medical model" approach to patients, reflecting their medical training and service requirements in multiple settings. This approach serves trainees well in many, if not most, clinical situations. While resident exposure to treatment of many psychiatric disorders will feel like a continuation of medical training (evidence driven, informed by treatment algorithms, oriented to "fixing" a symptom), residents' experiences with patients with personality disorder pathology will likely feel different, even disorienting, requiring additional, specific training. Residents face unique challenges in the management of patients with personality disorders. Regardless of whether personality disorder is the primary diagnosis or is co-occurring with other presenting conditions, patient management is greatly enhanced by perspectives that go beyond familiar medical paradigms.

Psychiatry residents are often the first responders in clinical situations involving patients with personality disorder (PD) symptoms. Long before psychiatry residents have begun training and practice in individual psychotherapy, they encounter patients with PD symptoms in emergency rooms, inpatient psychiatric services, and in consultation-liaison psychiatry on the medical floors. Often these patients are in crisis.

Practice trends in recent years underscore that patients seen in tertiary care settings often have unusually complicated presentations that can include personality disorder comorbidity [3]. These patients have typically "failed" standard treatments provided by primary care or mental health clinicians in the community, resulting in referral to tertiary centers where their primary providers are often trainees who see these patients across a variety of inpatient, emergency, and outpatient settings. Residents feeling competent treating primary mood, anxiety, or psychotic disorder patients can easily become overwhelmed or deskilled when treating PD patients. These feelings – of being overwhelmed, deskilled, or simply confused – are heightened when residents treat patients with PD pathology without an appreciation of the pathology or without an anchoring approach to assessment and treatment or, even worse, with a suspicion of the diagnosis and a prejudice against those with it.

Introducing residents to psychodynamic theory and providing them basic training in psychodynamic psychotherapy practice are two distinct, but at times overlapping, challenges that confront those working in residency education. The influence of psychoanalytically-informed psychodynamic psychotherapy on psychiatry training has waned in recent years, a change that is reflected in patterns of professional activity now reported by psychiatrists nationwide [4]. The ACGME requires that psychiatry residents learn a variety of psychotherapeutic interventions including cognitive-behavioral therapy, supportive psychotherapy, brief psychotherapy, and psychodynamic therapy [5]. However, while the ACGME continues to require training in psychodynamic psychotherapy, many trainees do not plan to practice psychotherapy of any kind, including psychodynamic psychotherapy, after completing training. Residency programs therefore are in the position of teaching psychodynamic theory and individual psychodynamic psychotherapy practice to trainees, many of whom have no intention of ever practicing psychodynamic psychotherapy, as they plan for career paths in pharmacotherapy, administration, or research.

Currently, exposure to psychodynamic theory and practice during residency is most often integrated into residents' requirement for training in individual psychotherapy [6]. This requirement often comes at a point in training well after residents have been working in acute settings including inpatient units, emergency rooms, and medical floors. Psychodynamic theory and practice may be taught to residents using multiple theories from a number of schools of thought, often reflecting the particular orientation of teachers and supervisors tasked with teaching dynamics at any particular residency training program. As a consequence, residents often leave training with the sense that psychodynamic work is amorphous and lacks a unifying structure. In addition, psychodynamic curricula and clinical supervision may emphasize theory and practice more suited to treating higher-functioning patients, remaining at a remove from the more impaired patient population most often seen by psychiatry residents.

Despite the significant burden of BPD (and other personality disorders) on mental health systems, patients, and families, residency training programs often fail to provide trainees with more than superficial exposure to available evidence-based treatments for personality disorders which include, in addition to TFP, dialectical behavior therapy (DBT) and schema-focused therapy (SFT) (primarily cognitive-behavioral), mentalization-based therapy (MBT) (like TFP, primarily psychodynamic), and good psychiatric management (GPM) (eclectic) [7–10]. This training gap fails to address the well-described need for clinician training and expertise in management of personality disorder pathology presenting across the mental health and medical treatment continuum [11]. In response, one leading personality disorder researcher has called for required psychiatric residency training on BPD psychopathology and therapies [12].

The "structural interview" developed by Kernberg, the cornerstone of the TFP approach to patient assessment, deliberately outlines the clinician's sequential roles of physician, psychiatrist, and psychodynamic psychotherapist [13]. In this interview, the clinician's goal is to evaluate possible active medical and psychiatric conditions first, before exploring the patient's level of personality organization and possible maladaptive personality traits. The psychiatry resident's developing identity closely mirrors this process; the resident has been trained first as a physician, using a "medical model" approach to diagnostic assessment, and then during residency the trainee develops the more specific psychiatric approach to assessment, although still hewing to the "medical model" in the early stages of training. After a thorough assessment of medical and psychiatric conditions, the resident trained in TFP will move on to systematic evaluation of the patient's personality organization. TFP training provides the requisite framework and skills that allow the resident to complete such an evaluation, which entails employing specific questions aimed to elucidate the patient's level of identity diffusion or consolidation, most prominent defensive processes used, and level of reality testing, all the while monitoring the three channels of communication – what the patient says, how the patient behaves, and how the resident feels.

Patients with personality disorder symptoms can induce unusually powerful feelings in clinicians, causing *all* clinicians, including and perhaps particularly trainees, to face increased risk management concerns at times when working with this population. Psychiatry residents, who may have had limited risk management education, are often faced with unusually complex clinical situations involving these patients. TFP training offers residents an increased sensitivity to personality disorder pathology coupled with a stress on monitoring countertransference reactions, which together can complement the standard, albeit limited, risk management education provided by most training programs [14].

8.2   TFP Training as an Overarching and Practical Psychodynamic Approach to Patient Care During Residency

- *TFP offers residents an overarching psychodynamic framework for patient care including, but not limited to, individual psychotherapy.*
- *TFP principles can be applied to multiple clinical settings underscoring for trainees the broad utility of a unified psychodynamic theory in their work.*
- *TFP is anchored by a focus on diagnosis, an orientation familiar to psychiatry residents from their medical training.*
- *TFP's roots as a psychiatric psychodynamic approach will resonate with psychiatry trainees.*
- *TFP's approach will correspond with the patients residents actually see.*

TFP was first developed as an individual psychotherapeutic treatment for patients with BPO, a category of personality disorders that includes the more narrowly defined BPD along with narcissistic, histrionic, schizoid, and other personality disorders. Since that time TFP has been used as a treatment for a variety of patient populations and in a variety of settings [15]. Despite its growing evidence base and broadening application, TFP remains a relatively specialized intervention and therefore may seem like an unlikely candidate for wider use in psychiatry residency training. However, pilot programs have demonstrated the utility of TFP training both as an overarching psychodynamic "toolbox" for residents in a variety of clinical settings and as an organizing set of principles for residents' training in psychodynamic psychotherapy.

TFP was developed to aid clinicians treating patients with BPD, patients known to be unusually challenging and often unresponsive to the standard pharmacotherapeutic and psychotherapeutic interventions available. Using TFP in psychiatry training is partly informed by a hypothesis that developing competence in the treatment of patients with severe personality disorder pathology can serve as a useful foundation for clinical work with other patient populations.

TFP is an approach anchored in diagnostic rigor, an orientation to patient care familiar to psychiatry trainees from their medical education. TFP may feel more familiar to residents, in this respect, than other psychodynamic approaches that do not privilege diagnostic assessment as TFP does. The TFP approach to patient assessment, reflected in the structural interview, requires a stepwise assessment of symptom inventories followed by an equally detail-focused exploration of personality organization markers. While clinicians of multiple backgrounds and disciplines have contributed to the development of TFP, critical elements of the treatment include a specifically *psychiatric* perspective. This perspective, as reflected in the structural interview process, should feel neither alien nor alienating to psychiatry trainees, as it is at once psychodynamic and medical in its approach while focusing on descriptive features of psychopathology and personality functioning.

Research confirms that high numbers of patients seen in settings where psychiatry residents spend much of their training, such as inpatient psychiatry units, emergency rooms, and outpatient general psychiatry clinics, have significant personality disorder pathology [16–18]. Despite the high rates of personality disorder diagnoses in both community samples and treatment samples, psychiatry residency programs tend to focus on those disorders treated primarily with pharmacotherapy or what used to be called "Axis I" disorders. The outcome can be a disconnect of sorts – residents are taught about certain psychiatric disorders (e.g., mood, anxiety, or psychotic disorders) but often find themselves responsible for the care of patients with prominent personality pathology without much, if any, specific training. An all too familiar example is the patient with the dysphoria of characterological depression of BPD treated unsuccessfully over time by a resident with standard medications and therapies for a primary depressive disorder. Patients with what were previously described as "Axis I" conditions, such as Major Depressive Disorder, often have a comorbid personality disorder. Research has shown that treating *only* the "Axis I" disturbance, without addressing the personality disorder, often leads to limited treatment response or even treatment failure. On the other hand, proactive treatment of the personality disorder can facilitate concurrent treatment of a mood, anxiety, or other more clear-cut symptom [19]. A benefit of exposure to TFP training would be the requisite investigation of aspects of personality organization as part of the diagnostic assessment. The resident appreciative of the patient's personality pathology would have a radically different experience treating the BPD patient complaining of dysphoria, for example, than the resident ignorant of the BPD diagnosis.

Dr. U. Works at a Day Treatment Program as a Resident Where the Staff Avoids Making Personality Disorder Diagnoses to the Detriment of the Patients

Clinical vignette: Dr. U. is a first-year psychiatry resident assigned to work at a day program for college-aged patients. The day program sees a number of patients referred by the student health service at a nearby large state university. Dr. U. is asked to see a number of patients attending groups at the program, almost all of whom have been given primary mood or anxiety disorder diagnoses. Dr. U. is anxious to make a good impression

(continued)

(continued)

and feels it would be impertinent to question the diagnoses made by the day program staff, but she quickly finds the patients assigned to her care to be highly unreliable, often canceling or not showing for appointments, or dishonest, misusing medications prescribed or denying substance use but testing positive on urine toxicology screens for cannabis. During her year working at the day program Dr. U. often feels incompetent; in one particularly trying episode, the day program's director reprimands Dr. U. after he is contacted by a participant's parents who complain that Dr. U. "can't seem to get the medications right" for their non-compliant, cannabis-using daughter's putative "depressive" disorder.

During her third year of residency, Dr. U. is introduced to the concept of the structural interview and consideration of personality disorder pathology beyond the nosology of the DSM-5 categories. In this process Dr. U. recognizes that a number of the patients she had seen at the day program likely had primary or co-occurring personality disorder pathology, specifically borderline and narcissistic traits often with circumscribed elements of passive sociopathy. In this process Dr. U. also begins to reconsider her prior feelings of incompetence, now seeing this countertransference reaction as reflective of the dyad of suffering patient and uncaring or incompetent clinician alternating with a dyad of indifferent patient and devalued novice clinician. Dr. U. also begins to appreciate how, in retrospect, she found herself treating patients with personality disorder pathology without the benefit of a treatment contract and frame that might have helped address the patients' devaluing and dishonest behaviors.

Take Home Point: Psychiatry trainees can and should feel competent to make personality disorder diagnoses when appropriate.

8.3   TFP Training Is Applicable to Residents' Experience in Multiple Settings During Training

- *TFP principles can be of use to residents even before they begin their training as individual psychotherapists.*
- *TFP principles can be useful even when the resident does not have a clearly established relationship with the patient, as in acute care settings.*
- *TFP principles provide residents with a diagnostic evaluation process complementary to DSM-5 descriptive categories of personality pathology.*
- *TFP can help residents understand how personality disorder symptoms arise in acute settings and how to employ dynamically informed de-escalation interventions.*

One novel academic pilot program for TFP training during residency was developed with a goal, among others, of establishing for residents a useful and applicable treatment model to be used in acute care settings [1]. The premise of this program was that because TFP is both an evidence-based and diagnosis-focused psychodynamic treatment, it would be familiar to and "user-friendly" for psychiatry residents. The hypothesis was that while the TFP manual describes an intensive individual psychotherapy in detail, the "knowledge, attitude, and skills" associated with the treatment would be of use to psychiatry residents in their work with patients in other settings as well.

This pilot program introduces TFP principles sequentially over the residents' second, third, and fourth years of training using a small group of clinician-educators as instructors and supervisors. Second-year residents are introduced to object relations theory and the key elements of personality organization. Third-year residents learn about structural interviewing, treatment planning, and contracting informed by the results of this type of assessment process. The introduction of TFP as a specific treatment intervention begins in the third year and is followed up by a year-long weekly fourth-year elective. This elective combines a group review of residents' videotaped psychotherapy sessions with continued didactic material using the TFP manual as a guide. The elective focuses on repeated practicing of the structural interview, generating treatment recommendations informed by the results of this interviewing process, and establishing and maintaining a treatment frame.

The central elements of TFP's application in acute care training settings include an openness to making a personality disorder diagnosis with incomplete information, a sensitivity to the three channels of communication and in particular how a patient acts and how the clinician feels, and the use of interventions informed by an object relations theoretical orientation with an emphasis on practicality and common sense. In acute care settings, residents will not likely have an established relationship with the patient involved, so using psychodynamic thinking and associated interventions is not routine.

The customary approach to diagnosis taught in training involves a "decision-tree" or symptom checklist intervention using DSM-5 diagnostic criteria for all disorders including personality disorders. This type of approach may be appropriate for the residents' outpatient clinic rotations where patients presumably are stable enough to participate safely in a multi-part evaluation. In acute care settings, however, residents are often required to see patients and make clinical decisions based on limited interviews, often with incomplete clinical data as well, and under circumstances in which patients and families are distressed.

The object relations understanding of severe personality pathology rests on an appreciation of highly maladaptive, "primitive," or splitting-based defenses and associated behaviors reflecting those underlying dynamics. The TFP approach can be of use to residents in acute care settings who encounter situations mediated by patients' active splitting, as in conveyance of "black and white thinking," or by their oscillating idealizing and devaluing experiences of others. This approach proceeds from (1) the diagnostic assessment and appreciation of personality pathology, to (2) management of countertransference, then to (3) identification of the dominant object relations dyad (interpersonal pattern or paradigm) in play, including the dyad emerging in the transference. Often in a crisis the emerging dyad includes a patient's powerful paranoid experience of the treater. Residents are trained to identify the dyad in play and its associated affect, describe this to the patient in an effort to convey understanding, and then attempt an empathic confrontation of the splitting-based operations in evidence. Residents able to distinguish between the frank paranoia of a psychotic illness, for example, and the paranoia, particularly in the transference, of personality pathology, would approach a paranoid patient in the acute care setting differently, depending on the diagnostic assessment.

Dr. G. Uses TFP Techniques in the Emergency Department to Manage Patients with Likely Personality Disorder Pathology

Clinical vignette: Dr. G., a fourth-year psychiatry resident with an interest in schizophrenia research, found his psychodynamic psychiatry training, which included classes over 2 years and supervised conduct of psychotherapy cases with a TFP-trained supervisor, of some interest but not likely to be important in his work going forward both as a researcher and as a psychiatry emergency room clinician.

One night in the emergency room when Dr. G. was the senior resident on call, he was asked by a junior resident

(continued)

(continued)

to see a patient who had walked in for assessment of "panic attack" symptoms who had become verbally abusive to the staff and had threatened a lawsuit if she were not released immediately. A review of the patient's record indicated that a similar event 6 months prior had led to an altercation between this patient and another patient, causing the staff to use sedating antipsychotic and anxiolytic medications to calm the patient, leading to an extended stay in an observation bed.

Dr. G. approached the patient with a mix of irritation and trepidation. Dr. G.'s review of the patient's previous ER visit and discussion with the junior resident supported preliminary consideration of a personality disorder, despite the patient's record's listing "major depression" as primary diagnosis and the patient's chief complaint of "panic attacks" symptoms. Dr. G.'s consideration of a personality disorder diagnosis prompted him to make a point of monitoring his countertransference and to take steps to avoid any intervention that might lead to escalation of the situation.

Dr. G. found the patient on a gurney, furious about having to wear a hospital gown, berating the beleaguered nurse trying to complete an assessment, and cursing her boyfriend whose threat to break up with her had led to her panic attack. Dr. G. approached the patient asking himself "What is the dominant object relation?" in a way that felt grounding, leaving him feeling armed with a systematic approach in contrast to feeling like an unskilled security guard brought in to quiet a patient down. He then reflected on the apparent role reversal at play; the patient feeling powerless and helpless had "turned the tables" as evidenced by a dyad including the powerless, cowering staff.

Dr. G. engaged the patient with the express purpose of putting the patient's experience into words, identifying

(continued)

the patient's chief symptoms of anxiety, and attempting to use confrontation to bring into the patient's awareness contradictory aspects of the patient's experience, one side dominating her subjective experience and the other expressed in her behavior. Dr. G. approached the patient calmly and proceeded to put her experience into words while communicating empathy with her situation: "I can see you are in distress about being here and worried about getting the help you need." The patient responded: "What a stupid thing to say! I'm being mistreated, my clothes were taken away, and no one is listening to me!" Dr. G. continued: "Yelling at the nurse isn't likely to help her complete her evaluation any more quickly; in fact it probably makes her feel pretty badly." The patient replied: "I don't care how she or anyone here feels!" Dr. G. attempted to empathically call attention to the role reversal expressed in the patient's treatment of the staff by answering: "I realize last time you were here you ended up staying much longer than was helpful; you may feel the staff failed you at that time. I can assure you now the staff is trying to be of help to you. You may be berating them to make sure they feel as badly as you do and I can see why you might do that."

Dr. G. was pleasantly surprised to see that his intervention, informed by a guess about the dyad being enacted, allowed the patient to calm down. Dr. G. reflected that calling into question the patient's dissociated paranoid experience of the staff helped avoid the kind of escalation that had marked the patient's last ER presentation.

Take Home Point: Psychiatry trainees can use TFP principles in multiple settings where they are likely to encounter patients with personality disorder pathology.

8.4 TFP Can Serve as an Organizing Approach to the Practice of Individual Psychotherapy

> • *TFP can offer residents a unifying psychodynamic approach to psychotherapy.*
> • *Initially developed as a psychotherapy for BPD, TFP may be a model for residents practicing psychotherapy with a heterogeneous patient population.*
> • *TFP prioritizes exploration of the transference, often a challenge for trainees.*
> • *Exposure to TFP extends residents' exposure to manualized, evidence-based psychotherapies and their research bases.*
> • *TFP assists residents in assessing and treating in psychotherapy the more impaired or chronic patients they are often assigned.*

A second pilot program offered a senior resident TFP elective with the goal of exposing trainees to an evidence-based psychotherapy, other than DBT, for patients with BPD [2]. This elective included both individual supervision of cases and a group supervision component where residents presented clinical material to a team of TFP supervisors. In a summary article, two participating residents and the residency program's director described the residents' unexpected conclusion: TFP training provided both specific skills for treating patients with BPD, and a broader set of skills applicable to assessing and treating a wider range of patients in psychodynamic psychotherapy.

In their review of this elective, the residents made the point that TFP introduced them to certain key elements: a unified theory for managing psychotherapy treatment, establishment and maintenance of a treatment frame, and work in the transference with concurrent appreciation of countertransference reactions. Because TFP's initial development was with BPD patients, training in TFP emphasized a focus on the treatment frame and transference conveyed in an explicit and direct fashion that the residents' more general psychodynamic psychotherapy training had not. It is understandable that psychiatry residents may not be oriented to the centrality of the treatment frame; most models of psychotherapy do not emphasize the treatment frame and its multiple functions to the extent that TFP does. Learning to engage patients in exploration of timeliness, payment, missed sessions, or the nature of their participation in treatment may be novel – particularly in settings where treatment is free or where treaters themselves do not personally bill patients such as in some resident clinics and Veterans Administration hospitals. Residents are often confused about whether it is even reasonable to first establish psychotherapy goals with a patient (Is it patronizing? Is it controlling? Does it thwart the exploratory process?) and then how to manage challenges to or deviations from the treatment frame (Is it unempathic or asking too much of the patient?).

Focus on the treatment frame often leads to exploration of the transference, since the frame channels the patient's relationship to the therapist. However, residents are typically reluctant to work in the transference for a number of reasons: focusing on the transference may seem somehow "self-centered" or it may feel too intimate; residents may have concerns that talking about the relationship may engender powerful feelings, including angry or eroticized reactions; residents may assume that "working in the transference" requires psychotherapy training beyond that offered in residency. The pilot program's results underscored that a focus on the treatment frame and attention to transference and countertransference are essential in clinical care, are not beyond the abilities of psychiatry residents, and are necessary for, but not limited to, work with severely personality disorder patients.

TFP training has the additional benefit of offering residents an introduction to the process of using a manual for individual psychotherapy treatment beyond behaviorally focused treatments. Exposure to a manualized, evidence-based psychodynamic psychotherapy provides residents with a systematic and unified description of psychotherapy techniques. In addition, a manualized approach confers a legitimacy that may be of particular importance to trainees steeped in today's evidence-favoring academic environment. Review of TFP's evidence base educates residents about patient selection, treatment outcome measures, and comparability to other psychotherapy interventions. The use of a specific psychodynamic treatment manual is in contrast with other less systematic and possibly more confusing introductions to psychotherapy, which may include exposure to multiple (and at times conflicting) theoretical orientations *or* psychodynamic theory presented as anecdotal "pearls" without a reliable and organized source that can be revisited.

In many training programs, clinicians involved in teaching psychotherapy to psychiatry residents come from a program's voluntary faculty [20]. These supervisors may be treating patients in an office setting or clinic where patients are relatively stable, working, or insured. In contrast, residents developing their skills as psychotherapists may see patients in settings where patients pay limited or no fees. This patient population may include those with limited resources, who are either unable or unwilling to work, or consciously or unconsciously motivated to pursue subsidized or free treatment. One unfortunate outcome of this common situation can be a discrepancy between the supervisor's point of reference and the resident's experience "on the ground." In this setting, supervisors may collude with residents in "underdiagnosing" patients or seeing patients as healthier or more high functioning than they actually are. TFP provides trainees a way of assessing certain lower-functioning personality disorder patients and a vocabulary for describing the way the patients' pathology presents in treatment. The comprehensive structural interview, for example, requires consideration of the patient's aggression, predominant defenses (repression-based vs. splitting-based), and superego functioning – all critical concerns when considering lower-level personality disorder pathology and elements of the "vocabulary" referenced. The attention to the treatment frame will bring these themes to the fore: the resident may be alert to evidence of aggression ("The patient asked for a late appointment as a favor but never showed up!"), splitting-based defenses ("Last week she told me I was the best resident she'd had; this week she stormed out when I wouldn't give her Valium"), or superego compromise ("He said he was paid up, but the clinic records show he has a 3 month balance"). The TFP approach to diagnosis and its focus on frame issues make overly optimistic thinking with certain patients less likely and as a result give residents the experience of having supervision for the patients they are actually treating and not patients they (or their supervisors) would prefer to treat.

Dr. L. Feels Frustrated in His Treatment of a Patient with Personality Disorder Pathology

Clinical vignette: Dr. H. was exposed to psychodynamic psychotherapy as a resident, finding the varied theoretical approaches described by different supervisors to be confusing and often seemingly unrelated to the kinds of cases he was seeing in the residents' clinic. Dr. H. found that the fallback, generic supportive psychotherapy he provided seemed to have little impact on his patients, and the sessions often felt boring; he began to wonder why psychotherapy would be part of a sophisticated medical training. In particular, Dr. H. felt frustration with the psychotherapy cases turned over year after year, the patients apparently making little progress, settled into a type of custodial treatment, absent identifiable goals.

As an attending psychiatrist, Dr. H. volunteered to supervise second-year residents in their long-term psychotherapy program. By this time, Dr. H. had been exposed to the central elements of TFP and felt application of TFP

(continued)

(continued)

principles appropriate to the residents' psychotherapy cases, given the high rates of primary or co-occurring personality disorder pathology in the trainee's caseloads.

Dr. H. begins supervision with a resident, Dr. L., who has been treating a middle-aged woman with "Persistent Depressive Disorder" for a year in weekly psychotherapy. Dr. L. finds himself uninterested in the treatment, frustrated by his patient's sporadic attendance, and dismayed, when she does attend, by her exclusive attention to the details of her ineffective antidepressant regimen and its side effects and by her pattern of monopolizing their time together. He reports that the patient's prior treater in the residents' clinic, now recently graduated, also found the treatment boring and frustrating.

Dr. H. introduces Dr. L. to aspects of the structural interview, encouraging Dr. L. to reflect on his patient's primary complaint (inability to move up at her job) as reflective of possible personality disorder pathology (narcissistic grandiosity coupled with a fragile sense of self-worth, making effective assertiveness difficult) rather than a mood disorder unresponsive to support and medication. Dr. H. helps Dr. L. develop a language with which to explore this diagnosis with his patient, encouraging Dr. L. to revisit his treatment contract with his patient, with a focus on issues of attendance and likely limitations of medication in helping the patient address her chief goals. Dr. L. is initially reluctant to revisit aspects of the treatment contract, telling Dr. H. his point of reference for conducting dynamic psychotherapy has been his own treatment, which has had limited explicit discussion of goals and no exploration of the treatment frame, as his own attendance had never been a problem.

(continued)

(continued)

Dr. H. encourages Dr. L. to pay particular attention to how he feels (devalued, powerless) and how the patient behaves (uncommitted, comfortable). Dr. L. is able to bring up to his patient her frequent lateness and absences, leading the treatment to becoming enlivened, both more interesting to Dr. L. and more useful to his patient, as she becomes more open to linking her behavior in therapy with her difficulties at work including issues of avoidance and subtle devaluation of the other.

Take Home Point: Psychiatry trainees can use TFP principles, including a focus on the three channels of communication and the use of the treatment-contracting process, to make the treatment more helpful for the patient and more interesting for the trainee.

8.5   TFP Training May Help Fulfill the Need for Residents' Education About Personality Disorders

- *Personality disorders are significantly represented in the settings where residents work.*
- *Education about PD pathology is often not commensurate with residents' exposure to these patients during training.*
- *TFP training is applicable to a wide range of PD patients beyond those with BPD.*
- *TFP incorporates a distinctly psychiatric perspective, something not part of all evidence-based treatments for personality disorders.*
- *Dissemination of TFP to a broader audience in residency training requires practical solutions to realistic impediments and limitations.*

Patients with personality disorder pathology are well represented in almost all psychiatric treatment settings, but they are particularly well represented in those settings where psychiatry residents spend much of their time. Psychiatry residents are required to rotate through inpatient psychiatry units, emergency departments, and outpatient psychiatric clinics where surveys indicate patients with PD pathology represent a very significant portion of the patient population. One study done in an urban inpatient sample found that nearly 50 % of participants met criteria for BPD on semi-structured interview, while a retrospective chart review at a university-based clinic yielded rates of BPD trait or disorder of 22 % [21, 22].

Despite the irrefutable presence of significant numbers of patients with personality disorders in training settings, many residency programs have relatively limited didactic focus on the subject [23]. In a recent survey on resident didactic education in BPD, about half of programs responding described a specific didactic course on BPD, taught by an almost equal mix of full-time and clinical faculty, but about half of training programs responding did not offer any specific coursework in BPD, providing BPD didactic material in other general courses offered. The most commonly reported therapeutic technique in this survey was DBT. The authors questioned whether didactic training in BPD was sufficient, given BPD's prevalence rate. Limited didactic coverage can leave much of the education about personality disorders to clinical supervisors, who may or may not be interested in the subject of personality disorders or in psychotherapeutics. In this setting, management strategies often overemphasize the role of medication, the modality most familiar to residents and the attendings who supervise them. In contrast, the American Psychiatric Association Practice Guideline for Patients with Borderline Personality Disorder endorses psychotherapy, not medications, as the central element of treatment for this disorder [24].

The reality is that psychiatry residents assess and treat patients with personality disorder pathology throughout their training without exception. While residents can relatively easily master treatment algorithms for most disorders, treating PD patients requires additional training with supplemental support. Much of the standard material introducing residents to psychodynamic psychotherapy describes the need for a focus on the treatment frame and maintenance of boundaries but does not offer specific modifications for psychotherapeutic intervention based on severity of illness [25]. This presents particular difficulties for the treatment of patients with moderate to severe personality disorder pathology. In fact, trainees often find themselves flummoxed as they use a set of interventions developed for treatment of higher-functioning patients, informed by traditional ego psychology theory, with these patients. Without a specific focus on diagnosis and diagnosis-guided treatment, trainees often find themselves addressing more escalating personality pathology with increased overt support – sometimes with untoward outcomes that involve the resident in the pathology. Psychiatry residents may be, as many psychiatrists in practice are, reluctant to make a personality disorder diagnosis, often with unfortunate consequences. Introduction of TFP in training can be an accessible way for residents to become comfortable recognizing PD pathology and engaging patients in a useful and productive way.

TFP's application to a broader range of patients beyond those with BPD may be another benefit of its introduction in training. TFP's essential elements, including its diagnostic approach, the establishment and maintenance of a treatment frame, a focus on the dominant affect in both patient and therapist (i.e., attention to transference/countertransference), and the exploration of emerging object relations "paradigms," including those in the transference, are applicable to a treatment of a wide range of patients. Familiarity with these essential elements confers on trainees a sense of having a "road map" to use in treatment. This "road map" is useful for those patients with PD presentations not fully captured in DSM-5 nosology or those with subsyndromal presentations who have symptoms that fall below the DSM-5 cutoff.

Some other evidence-based treatments for personality disorders do not originate from a psychiatric perspective and may cause psychiatry trainees to feel somehow marginalized in their practice. These treatments may presuppose that the psychiatrist's role is that of "psychopharmacologist," limited to prescribing and not necessarily involved in the diagnostic assessment process or psychotherapy. Exposure to this approach may leave psychiatry residents feeling that, in fact, treatment of personality disorders should be left to other clinical specialties.

While TFP may provide a succinct and useful approach to the gap in residency training about personality disorders, its broader implementation requires careful consideration and strategizing. One residency training director, in a useful commentary on the senior elective TFP pilot program, outlined the multiple challenges in offering TFP at her location [26]. These challenges included (1) the varying attitudes about psychodynamic psychotherapy training at the many hospital sites where residents rotate, (2) some residents' limited enthusiasm for learning psychodynamic theory and practice, given their likely career trajectories, (3) the reality that mastery of key elements of psychodynamic psychotherapy cannot be achieved quickly or easily, and (4) the lack of local TFP supervisors and the likely need for off-site supervision to complement available faculty at many programs.

Despite these concerns, this commentary underscored the potential benefits of introducing TFP as a general way to teach psychodynamic theory and practice that would interest skeptical residents and prove useful throughout their training. Training programs with limited resources might introduce the TFP model through (1) assignment of one supervisor to oversee a 3-year TFP curriculum, (2) use of group supervision for introduction of TFP concepts throughout training, (3) reliance on the TFP manual to reinforce essential concepts, and (4) ongoing training and supervision of local faculty done via Skype with off-site TFP-trained instructors. The International Society for Transference-Focused Psychotherapy's (ISTFP) standardized curriculum for TFP, in its abbreviated format, could serve as a useful template for residency training programs [27].

Dr. S. Works with a Patient with Narcissistic Personality Disorder Traits and Uses the Structural Interview Process to Broaden His Appreciation of Personality Pathology Diagnoses

Clinical vignette: Dr. S. is a psychiatry resident working at an intensive outpatient program (IOP) during his second year of training. In his residency curriculum thus far, Dr. S. has learned about personality disorders in one 45-minute overview of DSM-5 criteria with some discussion of epidemiology and one 45-minute lecture by a psychologist running a DBT skills group attended by some of the IOP patients.

Dr. S. is assigned to evaluate a 30-year-old man who has had almost 5 years of treatment for "depression" with essentially no response. This patient is college educated but has been unemployed since graduation, living with his parents who have used some of their retirement savings to pay for their son's treatment. Dr. S. is struck in his assessment of a total absence of neurovegetative symptoms in this patient's history. While the patient describes feeling "terrible" and unable to move forward in either meaningful work or an active social life, he reports generally good sleep, appetite, energy, and libido. On additional questioning, the patient describes to Dr. S. his marked sensitivity to rejection, his concern that any job he might take would be "beneath him" as he had graduated from a prestigious college, and his hopes that classes at a local acting school might lead to opportunities in the film industry.

Dr. S. presents this case in the IOP's daily rounds. Colleagues suggest additional antidepressant medication trials, but Dr. S. notes his patient has already had all of those mentioned. There is some consideration of recommending this patient attend the DBT skills group, but Dr. S. notes that the patient evinces essentially no BPD traits. When Dr. S. presents the case in the IOP's weekly meeting

(continued)

(continued)

with a consultant, a discussion of the structural interview approach leads to consideration of the patient's level of organization. Dr. S. finds discussion of the patient's lack of identity consolidation, use of primitive defenses, and passive dependence on his parents for support to be resonant. Dr. S. finds the concept of a "thin-skinned" narcissistic patient to be helpful, as the DSM-5 criteria for narcissistic personality disorder do not easily apply to his patient. When reading further, Dr. S. finds the structural interview's "dimensional" element to be a useful concept, explaining his patient's global impairment and providing Dr. S. with helpful "shorthand" for assessing personality pathology.

Take Home Point: The psychiatry resident's ability to assess for personality disorder pathology, including but not limited to DSM-5 categories, can add a dimension to the process of diagnosis.

8.6 The Structural Interview's Deliberate Approach to Diagnosis Should Be of Use to Residents

- *The structural interview approach fits well with the resident's training in succession as physician, psychiatrist, and psychodynamic psychotherapist.*
- *The structural interview supports the resident's obligation to master standard descriptive psychiatry and anticipates the DSM-5 appendix "hybrid" personality disorder model.*
- *The structural interview process can correct an approach to diagnosis that minimizes the contribution of personality disorder pathology.*
- *The structural interview helps residents in determining the psychotherapy best suited to a specific patient.*

The structural interview informs the patient assessment process in TFP in a manner at once flexible and focused. This approach requires a deliberate and systematic investigation first of medical or organic contributions to a patient's chief complaint, followed by clarification of any contribution of psychiatric illness (what were previously described as Axis I disorders), before an investigation of personality organization. This process closely mirrors the professional development of the psychiatric resident and should feel more familiar than a psychodynamic assessment process divorced from a standard medical orientation.

The structural interview begins with open-ended questions about why the patient is seeking treatment and how he understands his problem; the patient's response may immediately cue the interviewer to refine his questioning if it seems that a primary organic or medical disorder might be at hand. This refined questioning may include detailed exploration of a patient's mentation, including alertness, orientation, and memory. The resident using this approach may conclude from evidence of active impairment in basic cognitive functioning that a patient requires a thorough medical or neurological assessment before additional investigation. For the patient without a clear medical or organic process in evidence, the resident's next focus would be on possible primary psychiatric disturbances including mood, psychotic, or anxiety disorders. The psychiatry resident will be well versed in the DSM-5 diagnostic nosology and the questioning directly correlated to the diagnostic criteria of these categories.

The structural interview includes discussion of the DSM-5 category diagnostic criteria, including those for the personality disorders, and adds assessment of dimensional elements of a patient's presentation and functioning, such as understanding of self and of interpersonal functioning. In this way the structural interview closely resembles the alternative hybrid categorical-dimensional approach in the DSM-5 Section III appendix. A resident familiar with the structural interview approach to personality disorder pathology would find the essential concepts of this new, alternative approach familiar [28].

Use of the structural interview approach in training would correct for any pattern of avoiding exploration of personality disorder pathology a resident might develop over time. In the past, this phenomenon was often reflected in residents' notes reading: "Axis II – deferred." Residents may feel too inexperienced to confidently make personality disorder diagnoses, especially if their supervisors convey a reluctance to do so themselves. Use of the structural interview makes minimization of personality organization exploration impossible and gives residents a vocabulary to describe elements of personality organization absent from DSM-5 terminology.

The structural interview gives trainees a "shorthand" of sorts to use when making decisions about what kind of psychotherapy, if any, might benefit a patient. Use of a TFP approach to assessment does not automatically lead to a recommendation for TFP as a treatment. The structural interview provides residents with a way to think beyond a generic, unfocused recommendation for "therapy," given its deliberate approach. Is the patient's chief complaint related to a primary medical concern? Does it therefore make sense to recommend a supportive psychotherapy? If the patient's primary diagnosis is a psychiatric one (obsessive-compulsive disorder, anorexia nervosa), is a referral to a behavioral therapy with a strong evidence basis preferred? When considering a referral to a psychodynamic psychotherapy for personality disorder symptoms, the resident versed in the structural interview process will have some sense of prognostic indicators. Do the results of the structural interview indicate a likely positive response to exploratory treatment (relative identify consolidation, absence of obvious antisocial traits, capacity to use early interpretations)? Or does the interview suggest "red flags" for a psychodynamic psychotherapy referral, such as persistently impaired reality testing, limited capacity for abstract thinking, or evidence of "secondary gain" only as motivation?

Dr. Q. Is Asked to Evaluate a Patient and Initiate Treatment Without a Clear Sense of the Patient's Diagnosis

Clinical vignette: Dr. Q. is a resident assigned to work at her department's day treatment program. Ms. W., the social worker in charge of intakes, asks Dr. Q. to see a patient, Ms. M., whom Ms. W. has evaluated for possible combined individual psychotherapy and management of medications "as soon as possible." Ms. W. has concluded from her evaluation that the prospective patient, a graduate student, has "attention deficit disorder" and a depressive disorder. Ms. W. surmises that Ms. M.'s attention and mood difficulties have contributed to her difficulties at the office where she is assigned, resulting in placement on probation because of sloppy work.

Dr. Q. reviews Ms. W.'s notes and is interested to read that Ms. M. had a pattern of falling asleep during therapy session with her prior treater. Ms. W. did not investigate this further but in discussion did mention to Dr. Q. that Ms. M. had appeared to doze off during their evaluation, which she ascribed to her long hours at work and occasional cannabis use.

Dr. Q. approaches her evaluation with Ms. M. with the structural interview process in mind. She begins by reviewing with Ms. M. her symptoms of falling asleep abruptly and clarifies to what extent this has been assessed. Ms. M. reports she is awaiting sleep study results but conveys to Dr. Q. an urgency to start "therapy" as soon as possible given her poor performance at work. Dr. Q. is aware that despite the pressure she feels from Ms. W. and Ms. M., she needs to have any potentially treatment- interfering medical or psychiatric symptoms fully evaluated before beginning any kind of psychotherapy treatment. Dr. Q. is not sure what Ms. M.'s excessive daytime somnolence might reflect – a primary sleep disturbance, narcolepsy, or intoxication – but she

(continued)

(continued)

feels confident that this symptom requires exploration before she can make a commitment to psychotherapy.

Dr. Q. tells Ms. W., "I don't know what Ms. M.'s symptom reflects. I do know that it is important first to rule out any medical condition that might have a negative impact on her treatment. If it isn't narcolepsy, then I'll have to investigate whether it reflects active intoxication and I can do that by toxicology screen. If the problem is insomnia, we'll need to address that too; I understand the urgency in beginning treatment, but being able to stay awake is a requirement." Ms. W. reiterates her sense of urgency that Ms. M. begin "therapy" because of the crisis situation, but Dr. Q. stands by her approach to proceed in a stepwise manner to insure in advance that any psychotherapy she might offer would be the appropriate treatment and one the patient could participate in fully.

Take Home Point: Psychiatry residents can and should proceed methodically with the process of clinical diagnosis and use their medical knowledge and understanding of standard psychiatric diagnoses as is expected in the structural interview.

8.7 TFP Principles Assist Residents with Risk Management

- *Psychiatry residents receive limited formal risk management training.*
- *PD pathology is often associated with common risk concerns.*
- *Training status is associated with particular risk vulnerabilities with PD patients.*
- *TFP's focus on frame and countertransference are useful risk management tools.*

Formal risk management training in psychiatry residency is limited, and much of the risk management education residents receive is done "ad hoc," often with faculty offering anecdotal evidence to guide decision-making. Specific risk management training related to treating PD patients is rare, although it is common sense to assume that while all clinicians face unusually challenging situations with PD patients, residents in particular are vulnerable in this context.

Experts in medicolegal issues in psychiatry focus on those areas associated with the most common types of malpractice claims: incorrect treatment, suicide/attempted suicide, drug reactions, incorrect diagnosis, unnecessary commitment, and undue familiarity [29]. While clinicians may be sued in the course of treating patients with *any* diagnosis, a review of this list suggests the particular risks associated with treating patients with PD pathology. Residents may be particularly vulnerable given their relative inexperience, likely emphasis on "going the extra mile" for patients, concerns about limit setting or being perceived as "mean" by patients, or bias toward providing any and all services to a patient in crisis.

For residents treating patients with BPD, the combination of the patient's particular pathology and the residents' relative inexperience can be concerning. The risk management concerns well described in treating BPD – such as over-involvement leading to unnecessary treating, including pharmacotherapy or hospitalizations, or a countertransference of anger, or sadism leading to distancing or abandonment – may be increased for trainees [30, 31].

TFP training offers a particular and specific focus on frame and countertransference matters. Attention to the frame can help residents monitor their own over-involvement, such as allowing sessions to go longer than scheduled or "heroic" dedication leading to late evening or weekend meetings with patients. The TFP focus on countertransference can help trainees monitor themselves for excessive identification with or devotion to a patient or conversely hateful feelings that could contribute to inattention to serious matters [32]. The TFP approach to the suicidal patient can help residents avoid assuming a role as the patient's "savior" and allow them to feel free to have after-hour safety assessments done in the emergency department rather than on the phone when the resident is without supervision. TFP principles applied to prescription practices, including monitoring a countertransference reaction to "fix" the patient with yet another medication or provide the patient with a larger than usual dose or supply of medication to address the patient's distress, would be another useful risk management element. TFP's endorsement of frank discussion of a patient's PD diagnosis with the patient helps trainees avoid the precarious situation of documenting one diagnosis (say, BPD) but describing to the patient and family another diagnosis (say, treatment-resistant depression). Such a pattern of "keeping two sets of books" could present a serious risk management issue if there were an untoward event.

Certain commonly seen dyads may be of additional risk for residents. For example, one familiar dyad and its inverse is the BPD patient who feels herself to be on the receiving end of cruel and hurtful behavior (such as when a resident attempts to maintain a treatment frame with limits on length of session or intersession contact), alternately with the patient's sadistic acting out (threatening to report the resident to his training director for misbehavior), leading the trainee to feel shamed and paralyzed. The TFP approach involving identification of dyads including those in the transference can bring into the residents' awareness potentially compromising situations, thereby allowing for changes in behavior to avoid patterns that would increase risk.

Dr. R. Makes Exceptions for Her Patient, Leading to a Series of Potentially Compromising Situations

Clinical vignette: Dr. R. is a second-year resident assigned to treat Ms. P., a woman in her mid-20s with an extensive history of anxiety and depression symptoms. Dr. R. is a

(continued)

(continued)

highly conscientious clinician who distinguished herself during internship for her unusual commitment to her clinic patients.

Ms. P. lives with her parents, works part-time (well below her level of education), and has few friends. Ms. P. often tells Dr. R. of her passive suicidality, given that none of the many medications she has tried has addressed her long-standing feelings of emptiness and lack of direction. Dr. R. sometimes wonders if Ms. P. may have personality disorder traits along with her mood and anxiety symptoms, but she is cautioned by her clinic supervisor to put off making a PD diagnosis until the other symptoms have remitted.

Ms. P. reports to Dr. R. that sleep/wake cycle reversal makes it difficult to come to appointments until after 5 pm when the clinic is closed. Dr. R. agrees to meet with Ms. P. after hours, given her concern about Ms. P.'s persistent symptoms and apparent intractable insomnia. Over time Ms. P. asks Dr. R. for appointments even later in the evening; Ms. P. tells Dr. R. their appointments "are the only thing that make life worth living," causing Dr. R. increasing guilt about her impulse to set a limit on the after-hours meetings. During their meetings Ms. P. alternates between declaring her appreciation, which Dr. R. finds gratifying, and voicing her persistent hopelessness and suicidality, which Dr. R. finds unnerving.

When Dr. R. is assigned a new supervisor in her third year, she is reluctant to tell Dr. C. the details about her treatment with Ms. P., although she does so with some chagrin. Dr. C. uses this opportunity to review with Dr. R. her thinking about Ms. P.'s diagnosis and to encourage her to revisit with Ms. P. the frame for their treatment. Dr. R. describes to Dr. C. her concern that a frame with more clear limits would lead Ms. P. either to anger with Dr. R. or to despair with increased suicidality. With support

(continued)

(continued)

from her supervisor, Dr. R. is able to introduce to Ms. P. the possibility of a contribution of a personality disorder diagnosis to her active symptoms and to revise their treatment frame so that they meet only when the clinic is open. This discussion allows Ms. P. to express to Dr. R. that setting a limit on the time of their meetings felt to her as though Dr. R. did not really care about her anymore. Dr. R. was able to tolerate this conversation, cognizant of Ms. P.'s ability to engage Dr. R. with omnipotent control, as well as the patient's alternating idealization and devaluation of Dr. R. as it related to aspects of the treatment frame. Dr. R. is able to hear Dr. C.'s caution about the risks associated with over-involvement and ways attention to the treatment frame can keep that in check.

Take Home Point: Use of the structural interview and elucidation of personality disorder pathology is good risk management technique, particularly necessary for the trainee who is uncertain about her skills.

References

1. Zerbo E, Cohen S, Bielska W, Caligor E. Transference-focused psychotherapy in the general psychiatry residency: a useful and applicable model for residents in acute clinical settings. Psychodyn Psychiatry. 2013;41(1):163–81.
2. Bernstein J, Zimmerman M, Auchincloss E. Transference-focused psychotherapy training during residency: an aide to learning psychodynamic psychotherapy. Psychodyn Psychiatry. 2015;43(2):201–22.
3. Bladder JC. Acute inpatient care for psychiatric disorders in the United States, 1996 through 2007. Arch Gen Psychiatr. 2011;68(12):1276–83.
4. Olfson M, March SC, Pincus HA. Trends in office-based psychiatric practice. Am J Psychiatr. 1999;156(3):451–7.

5. Mellman LA, Beresin E. Psychotherapy competencies: development and implementation. Acad Psychiatry. 2003;27(3):149–53.
6. Gastelum E, Douglas CJ, Cabaniss DL. Teaching psychodynamic psychiatry to psychiatry residents: an integrated approach. Psychodyn Psychiatry. 2013;41(1):127–40.
7. Linehan MM. Dialectical behavioral therapy for borderline personality disorder. New York: Guilford; 1992.
8. Young JE, Klosko JS, Weishaar ME. Schema therapy: a practitioner's guide. New York: Guilford; 2003.
9. Bateman A, Fonagy P. Effectiveness of partial hospitalization in the treatment of borderline personality disorder: a randomized controlled trial. Am J Psychiatr. 1999;156(10):1563–9.
10. McMain SF, Links PS, Gnam WH, Guimond T, Cardish RJ, Korman L, Streiner DL. A randomized trial of dialectical behavioral therapy versus general psychiatric management for borderline personality disorder. Am J Psychiatr. 2009;166(12):1365–74.
11. Biskin RS, Paris J. Management of borderline personality disorder. Can Med Assoc J. 2012;184(17):1897–902.
12. Gunderson JC. Borderline personality disorder: ontogeny of a diagnosis. Am J Psychiatr. 2009;166(5):530–9.
13. Kernberg OF. Severe personality disorders. New Haven: CT Yale University Press; 1984.
14. Simon RI, Shuman DW. Therapeutic risk management of clinical-legal dilemmas: should it be a core competency? J Am Acad Psychiatr Law. 2009;37:155–61.
15. Yeomans FE, Clarkin JF, Kernberg OF. Transference-focused psychotherapy for borderline personality disorder: a clinical guide. 1st ed. Washington, DC: American Psychiatric Publishing; 2015.
16. Zimmerman M, Rothschild L, Chelmininksi I. The prevalence of DSM-IV personality disorders in psychiatric outpatients. Am J Psychiatr. 2005;162(10):1911–8.
17. Widiger TA, Rogers JH. Prevalence and comorbidity of personality disorder. Psychiatr Ann. 1989;19:132–6.
18. Widiger TA, Weissman MM. Epidemiology of borderline personality disorder. Hosp Community Psychiatr. 1991;42:1015–21.
19. Gunderson JG, Stout RL, Shea MT, Grilo CM, Markowitz JC, et al. Interactions of borderline personality disorder and mood disorders over 10 years. J Clin Psychiatr. 2014;75:829–34.
20. Clemens NA, Notman MT. Psychotherapy and psychoanalysts in psychiatric residency training. J Psychiatr Pract. 2012;18:438–43.

21. Sansone RA, Songer DA, Gaither GA. Diagnostic approaches to borderline personality disorder and their relationship to self-harm behavior. Int J Psychiatr Clin Pract. 2001;5:273–7.

22. Sansone RA, Rytwinski D, Gaither GA. Borderline personality disorder and psychotropic medication prescription in an outpatient psychiatry clinic. Compr Psychiatr. 2003;44:454–8.

23. Sansone RA, Kay J, Anderson JL. Resident education in borderline personality disorder: is it sufficient? Acad Psychiatry. 2013;37(4):287–8.

24. American psychiatric association practice guideline for the treatment of patients with borderline personality disorder. Am J Psychiatr. 2001;159(suppl).

25. Gabbard GO. Long-term psychodynamic psychotherapy: a basic text. 2nd ed. Arlington, VA: American Psychiatric Publishing; 2014.

26. Chambers JE. Discussion of transference-focused psychotherapy training during residency: an aide to learning psychodynamic psychiatry. Psychodyn Psychiatry. 2015;43(2):223–8.

27. http://istfp.org/training/training-in-tfp/.

28. Oldham JM. The alternative DSM-5 model for personality disorders. World Psychiatr. 2015;14(2):234–6.

29. Hales RE, Yudofsky SC, Roberts LW. Textbook of psychiatry. 6th ed. Washington, DC: American Psychiatric Publishing; 2014.

30. Gutheil TG. Suicide, suicide litigation, and borderline personality disorder. J Pers Disord. 2014;18(3):248–56.

31. Gutheil TG. Borderline personality disorder, boundary violations, and patient-therapist sex: medicolegal pitfalls. Am J Psychiatr. 1989;146(5):597–602.

32. Winnicott DW. Hate in the counter-transference. Int J Psychoanal. 1949;30:69–74.

Index

© Springer International Publishing Switzerland 2016   267
R.G. Hersh et al., *Fundamentals of Transference-Focused
Psychotherapy*, DOI 10.1007/978-3-319-44091-0

Printed in the United States
By Bookmasters